CHILD SURVIVAL, HEALTH AND SOCIAL WORK INTERVENTION

About the Author

Dr. Sandhya Joshi is presently working as a Reader at Faculty of Social Work, M.S. University of Baroda, Baroda (India) and has more than 15 years of experience of teaching Social Work at post-graduate level. She obtained her master's degree from Delhi School of Social Work, University of Delhi and doctoral degree form M.S. University of Baroda. Recipient of Cleveland International Fellowship of one year, Dr. Joshi, inter alia, undertook research work at the Cuyahoga CountyDepartment of Children and Family Services, Cleveland, U.S.A. She has also presented professional papers on various subjects in India and abroad. Her special interest fields are social development, health and well being of women and children. She has actively associated herself with a few voluntary organisations in Baroda city.

CHILD SURVIVAL, HEALTH AND SOCIAL WORK INTERVENTION

DR. SANDHYA JOSHI
Reader
Faculty of Social Work
M.S. University
Baroda

CONCEPT PUBLISHING COMPANY PVT. LTD.
NEW DELHI-110059

The Indian Council of Social Science Research gave the financial support towards the publication of this work. However, the responsibility for the contents of the book — facts, opinions, conclusions, etc. — is entirely that of the author and not of the ICSSR.

ICSSR Consultant : **Prof. Rajeshwar Parsad**

ISBN: 978-81-7022-576-8

First Published 1996

Published and Printed by

Concept
Since 1974

Concept Publishing Company Pvt. Ltd.
A/15-16, Commercial Block, Mohan Garden,
New Delhi-110059 (India)
T : 91-11-41101460
E : publishing@conceptpub.com, *W*: www.conceptpub.com

"I soon can learn to do it,
If you'll let me see it done;
I can see your hands in action,
But your tongue too fast may run;
And the lectures you deliver
May be very fine and true.

But I'd rather get my lesson
By observing what you do,
For I may misunderstand you
And the high advice you give,
But there is no misunderstanding
How you act and how you live!"

— *Anonymous*

ACKNOWLEDGEMENTS

First and foremost, I wish to place on record my ever spontaneous and profound sense of gratitude towards my guiding teacher, Dr. (Mrs.) Promilla Maitra. It is no exaggeration when I state that I have always held Dr. Maitra in the highest esteem which one can have only for one's 'Professional ego ideal'. She not only motivated me to undertake experimental research (which is rather uncommon in Social Work discipline) but was always there when I needed her. It has indeed been a momentous experience to complete my studies under her erudite guidance. Next, I am heavily indebted to Dr. H.M. Rajyaguru, earlier a Reader at Faculty of Social Work, whom I used to consult every now and then for his expertise in Social Work Research Anytime I felt unsure regarding a technical matter he was the one who suggested the most convincing solutions. The present study would have been literally impossible without the continuous consultancy and logistics support extended so very kindly by Dr. Sagun Desai (Pharmacologist) and Dr. Anita Kothiala, (Paediatrician) both from Medical College, Baroda. Words fail me to express adequately the gratitude I feel towards Mr. J.C. Sharma, Reader and Incharge-EDP Section, Tata Institute of Social Sciences, Bombay for the consultancy in Statistics and electronic data processing provided by him in my work. I must also acknowledge the support provided by the Indian Council of Social Science Research for sanctioning me a research grant covering full cost of computerized analysis of my data at TISS, Bombay.

All through the period of my doctoral work, Mr K.M. Sharma, Mr. I.P. Shelat, Dr. I.M. Patel, Dr. H.M. Rajyaguru, Dr. V.N. Anjaria and Mr. S.B. Saxena have helped in numerous ways in their respective appointment of the Dean or the head of the Department at this faculty. I am sincerely grateful to them all. Similarly, my family members who had to face the worst whenever I was overworked and tired, must be thanked too. In fact, without the constant support and encouragement from my husband Col. S.M. Joshi and my sons Umang, Tarang this study might not have been complete in good time as it happens to be today.

Last but not the least my profuse thanks are due towards People who participated in the project.

SANDHYA JOSHI

CONTENTS

LIST OF TABLES

LIST OF FIGURES

1

INTRODUCTION

All over the world since the late seventies, the perspectives on health have undergone a revolutionary change. Contrary to the old paradigm of economic growth in which health was viewed as an item of consumption, health is now recognized as a critical commodity of investment for social development. At the Dag Hammerskjoeld Seminar at Uppasala in 1977 on "another Development in Health" it was categorically proclaimed, inter alia, that health is a human condition which cannot be delivered by medical services alone and the people have the right and duty to participate individually and collectively in the planning and implementation of health care services. In the context of the third world countries it was further stated that the existing system of hospital based services has failed to reach the masses and the strategies of organising community involvement in health programmes as well as achieving fundamental social and economic change were recommended emphatically.

Ideally, community involvement should mean that the initiatives come from the people in various forms including presenting proposals for improving health situation of people; translating these proposals into concrete plans; and implementing (evaluation follows) them with the necessary assistance from state or voluntary agencies. In reality, however, this rarely happens. In fact, in India, sometimes people also hesitate in coming forward voluntarily to participate in health camps, programmes or campaigns. This need not surprise anybody because people in general, lack technical knowhow, access to resources and they are unorganised (to be in a position to wield collective power). Yet, the people are known to extend their cooperation and participate when social workers or other professionals successfully motivate them. "Motivating people" here implies use of social work techniques (of working with people) to make them aware of their health needs; modify their attitudes towards health as a desirable goal; improve their health seeking behaviour; and finally encourage optimum and timely utilisation of available services by upgrading their knowledge, explaining procedures and removing other seeming hurdles.

Further to application of social work techniques in motivating people to utilise existing health services, one must consider their need and relevance in situation where the sources of health hazards have been directly traced to peoples' own behaviour on various accounts *viz.* superstitions and socio-cultural beliefs affecting health; lack of personal hygiene and environmental sanitation; faulty dietary habits; lack of knowledge regarding 'balanced meal' and 'nutritious recipes'; sex or age based biases in intra-family food distribution; social distance within a community which creates barriers like denial of access to safe drinking water; and helpless and dependent sections of the society like children and women to some extent. This also highlights the inadequacy of a narrowly technological approach to health issues and advocates for an interdisciplinary approach which takes due cognizance of utterly human dimensions at work in health concerns. It is in this context that the present field project of upgrading health of underfive slum children was taken up with the intent of working out an intervention module through a systematic application of professional social work knowledge and skills with valuable aid from medical and para medical professionals.

At this juncture, it is imperative to bring out the significance of our focus on child health, in particular. Health children can be the greatest resource of any country. More so for a developing country like India where children form a wide base of the population pyramid. As per Park J.E. and Park K. (1985 : 435) in India 17 per cent of the population comprises of children under 5 years and another 35 per cent in the range of 5 to 16 years. But it is not by sheer numbers alone that the advocates of comprehensive health care for the child population stress their point. The most crucial period in a child's life is the first five years during which about 40 per cent of physical and 80 per cent of mental growth and development occurs. In the case of poor children, malnutrition causing lowered resistance to various infections in early childhood can threaten their very survival. In case of malnutritioned underfives who do survive (The bouts of childhood killer diseases, namely, diptheria, tetanus, whooping cough, diarrhoea, polio, measles and pneumonia), various reports have indicated that they do not attain for several years the same nutritional status as the healthy children of well to do class of the same age or have to live with some form of disability. The association between malnutrition in the preschool children and low levels of mental performance has also been well documented in several regions of the world where malnutrition is highly prevalent.

In addition to protein energy malnutrition, the two other major health problems of pre-schoolers in India are vitamin 'A' deficiency and iron deficiency anaemia. In fact vitamin 'A" deficiency has been a major public health problem leading to xerophthalmia (nightblindness) in many developing countries. Severe form of this deficiency can cause permanent blindness and in India 20 per cent of cases of blindness have been attributed to it.

1.2 Health and Nutrition Status of Underfives in India

Major indicators of health and nutrition status of underfive children paint a grim scenario. The following statistics highlight the harsh reality in convincing terms:

* Underfives Mortality Rate (U5MR) is alarmingly high at 142 per 1000 live births per year. India ranks 38th in the descending order of 129 nations of the world according to their U5MR — only a few African and Asian countries are worse off.
* Infant Mortality Rate (IMR) is also very high at 94 per 1000 live births per year.
* Thirty per cent children are born with low birth weight (2500 grams or less) which is a strong determinant of survival. On this account, the country has achieved the dubious distinction of leading the group of 129 nations documented by UNICEF's State of the World Children Report 1992.
* Also, 61 per cent children between the age of 0-4 years are classified as being moderately and severely underweight and another 9 per cent as severely underweight.
* An average Indian child of 1-5 years receives only 810 kilo calories per day as against the Indian Council of Medical Research recommended daily allowance (RDA) of 1200 k cals. However, somewhat on favourable side, pre-school children on staple diet of cereals and pulses manage to meet the needs of proteins to near adequacy.
* Therefore, it has been recognized that Indian underfives suffer from primary energy malnutrition and secondary protein

deficiency. Overall, 80 per cent children suffer from varying degrees of growth retardation.

* Dietary intake of vitamin 'A' is around 100 mu grams per day as against RDA of 300 mu grams.
* Percentage of fully immunized children under one year as per UNICEF's 1992 report improved dramatically during the eighties.

Year	Vaccine			
	TB	DPT	Polio	Measles
1981	12	31	7	—
1990	97	92	93	87

Similarly, per centage of pregnant women immunized for Tetanus (protection) went up from 24 in 1981 to 7.7 in 1990.

While, the above table presents a positive development indicating control of major childhood morbidity diseases which at times led to mortality or disability, a new threat to health of adults and children has emerged in recent years. In India, HIV infection has become entrenched in urban areas of the four metropolis with infection rates as high as 70 per cent among some groups of prostitutes. This is a potential source of morbidity amongst their children.

* Use of ORT—a low-cost health technology in management of diarrhoea was reportedly only 13 per cent during 1990.

1.3 Determinants of Child Survival and Health

Survival of a child at birth depends primarily upon his/her own health which in turn is a determinate of—

(a) mother's health during pregnancy.
(b) neo-natal health care practices in the family.

Both (a) and (b) above are further dependent upon a large number of socio-cultural and behaviour factors which can be enumerated as per below :

* Pregnancy health care beliefs and practices.
* Purchasing power for adequate nutrition.
* Age at maternity
* Proper spacing between births.

* Birth order of the child.
* Access to and utilization of ante-natal and post-natal services.
* Education of parents; mother more particularly.
* Mother's knowledge and competence of child health care during normal times as well as during illness of the child.
* Practice of giving/discarding collostrum at neo-natal stage.
* Breast-feeding practices : cleanliness and duration in particular.
* Sterilised feeding bottles or utensils used for the child.
* Preventive immunization by mother and child.
* Prophylaxis against vitamin 'A' deficiency and anaemia.
* Faith in doctors and modern medicine.
* Access to and utilization of curative services.
* Timely supplementary feeding and weaning.
* A safe physical environment ensuring adequate shelter, potable water and environment sanitation.

In short, it can be seen that child survival and development is governed by socio-cultural and physical environment in which the child is born and brought up. Certainly these factors are in the domain of social sciences and professional social work has tremendous scope and potential in promoting child health.

1.4 Child Survival and Social Work Intervention

To "Intervene" is to enter an interacting system of relationships or to come between or among persons, groups, neighbourhoods or communities with the intent of helping them. Since primary concern of social work profession is people in life situations where they (the people) have to strike a balance between compulsions of their socio-cultural environment on one hand and their capacities to cope with on the other, the requisite "help" is rendered through application of professional methods and techniques. The professional values and the scientific body of knowledge equip the practitioner with the right skills and attitudes towards people in their situation and facilitate his/her helping role while working with human systems either in independent or collaborative action. A detailed discussion of the concept and related issue would be taken up in chapter two. At this juncture, it is however, logical to first derive the close link between social work intervention and child health concerns and then present the repertoire of relevant professional techniques.

The raison d'etre of designing modules of social work interventions for promoting child health and survival can be stated as follows :

1.4.1 *Socio-cultural and Behavioural Determinants*

Section 1.3 has clearly brought out how a large number of socio-cultural and behavioural determinants influence child survival in a critical way. Let us take few examples here. First, the crucial variable of mother's education by formal or non-formal means. Even when differences in income and residence are allowed for, the survival chances of a child born to a woman with four or more years of education are significantly greater than those of a child whose mother has never been to school. The reason for the strong correlation between the material education and child survival are : an educated mother is more likely to be confident enough to seek help when needed or in other words, her health-seeking behaviour is more favourable; more likely to be aware of choices before her; and she is also more likely to assert herself and assume control over what happens to her family. Second, consider the facts that underfives deaths happen to mothers who are younger than 18 or older than 35; or those who have had more than 4 children already; or the women who conceive within less than 2 years of the previous delivery.

1.4.2 *Transfer of Medical Technology to field*

Medical technologies and the prescriptions related to it emerge from medical science. No matter how sound a given medical specification is, it would not work automatically on its own in the field. Non-medical techniques like extension work or social work techniques are required for effective transfer of a technology from "lab to land". In the words of Kochar V. (1991 : 95): it is one thing to establish that a few drops of vitamin 'A' will protect children from blindness of a certain type but it is quite another task to make available these vitamin drops in every single of the five-lakh odd villages in the country and further it is still more complex to ensure that every child of a certain age group is actually given these drops as per specifications. Similar has been the case of under achievement in attaining family planning targets in the past 40 years or so when various simple and free technologies for fertility control have been available in the country.

Arguably, each health care programme is accompanied by a designated set of guidelines and manuals for programme implementation tasks and procedures. Though these are useful to some extent, they are not very comprehensive. Also, the complex dynamics of working with human systems defy any fixed formula of social work intervention. Social work interventions, in addition to professional skills and knowledge call for high levels of sensitivity, creativity and pragmatic imagination.

1.4.3 *Complexity of Child Survival Monitoring Process*

Monitoring of child survival and development is a complex process not only because of the multiplicity of factors influencing child survival but also because these factors vary at different levels. In the words of Murthy N. (1986 : 179), at the micro level, mother's health and her weight gain during pregnancy may be significant factors in determining birth weight of a child. At the household level, education of the mother, family income and practices such as food habits and intra family food distribution have a significant role in determining probability of child survival. At the village level, environmental conditions and access to medical care may be the influencing factors. At the national level, adequacy of food production and its proper distribution would be factors influencing child health.

1.4.4 *Poverty and Vulnerability*

Development programmes aimed at reducing poverty do not necessarily and automatically reach children or improve the environment in which they live and grow. In most countries, there is a relative neglect of the children of pre-school age, although they are vulnerable and an 'at-risk' group deserving special health care programme. The second intricating factor in this context is the low propensity of the poor to utilise existing resources. Chow N.W (1984) states that for most countries in the world today, poverty means the inability to lead a healthy physical existence. Persistent conditions of poverty produce certain incompetencies and also a sense of deprivation which further debilitate the poor in their hard struggle for a basic living. Such a handicapped start in life reduces the ability of the poor to benefit from available opportunities or make fullest use of developmental services, including the health services. Regarding underutilisation of heath services, in India there is an added dimension of superstitions, traditions and religious practices which many a time discourage people away from modern health technologies.

1.4.5 *At - risk Status of Underfives*

Relatively, it would have been much easier to conduct this study with slightly older school going children since some of the inputs were periodic height and weight check up; thorough medical check up; haemoglobin testing; monitoring vitamin and iron supplement treatment prescribed by doctors etc. However, ultimately we decided in favour of the underfives due to the following reasons proffered by Park J.E. & Park K. (1985 : 435).

(i) Large Numbers

Children under-five years constitute 15 to 20 per cent of the general population in the developing countries (about 17 per cent in India). By virtue of their large numbers they are entitled to a large share of health care.

(ii) High Mortality

Apart from infant mortality which is more than 100 per 1000 live births in the developing countries, the mortality in the age group 1 to 4 years is also very high, not less than 40 per 1000 live births as compared to 0.5 in a developed country like Sweden. In fact, 50 to 60 per cent of total deaths in developing countries occur in children under five as compared to only 5 per cent in the developed countries. The major causes of death in this group are malnutrition and infection both of which are preventable.

(iii) Morbidity

The common diseases which affect the pre-school age group are Diptheria, Whooping cough, Diarrhoea, Dysentry, Skin infections, malnutrition, accidents—all preventable.

(iv) Growth and Development

The pre-school age period is a period of rapid growth and development. Since healthy children are the greatest resource of any country their growth and development needs monitoring.

(v) Accessibility

Infants and young children (1-4 years) are hard to reach. Special inputs are needed to bring the child into the orbit of special health care. Operational research all over the world has demonstrated that patients are unlikely to travel more than 5 to 8 km. to receive medical care. For the toddler who needs to be carried, this distance may be reduced even further.

1.5 Repertoire of Relevant Interventions

In the light of the discussion above social work interventions directed towards removal of socio-cultural barriers/reducing their malfeasance; affecting favourable attitudinal and behavioural changes; facilitating effective transfer of medical technologies to ground level; cutting through the complexities of child health monitoring processes; and providing special package of services needed by the vulnerable and at-risk children can be summarised as follows :

Mobilizing parents and health providers; social advocacy; improving communications between target group and component sections of the health system; improving communication abilities of the client system; working out forward and backward linkages between systems; programme organization; training of health workers and volunteers; counselling; child-to-child programmes; capacity building and empowering of people; promoting cost-effective health technologies; non-formal health education; community education and involvement; resource management etc.

1.6 Objectives of the Project

The broad objective was to construct, test, validate and document an alternate, neighbourhood based viable social work intervention model which could demonstrate measurable improvement in health and growth of underfive children belonging to an urban slum community by means of conducting a field experiment research.

The specific objectives for sake of enhanced clarity need to be presented separately for the base line survey and each of the input variables that were woven into the study design. Please refer Fig 1.1 to locate the relative positions of these variables in the total interventional process.

1.6.1 *Objectives of Baseline Survey*

(a) To identify experimental families *i.e.*, those families which had at least one child under the age of four years and three months (so that the child does not cross the age of five years before completion of the planned interventions) at the time of interviewing.

(b) To document socio-economic background *viz.*, language, caste, religion and migration particulars, family size, educational and occupational status of family members, economic condition, housing, environment and access to basic amenities.

(c) To study the food consumption levels and normal diet pattern of the family through recall method of 48 hours.

(d) To study utilization of health services affecting growth and well being of underfives *viz.* ante natal care, post natal care, family planning; trained attendance at delivery.

(e) To detect latent or hidden disabilities amongst experimental children below thirty months of age by administering Bailey's developmental testing tool.

1.6.2 *Objectives of Health Care and Growth-monitoring Package for Children (denoted as input A in Fig I.1)*

(a) To organise a thorough medical examination of treatment and control group children before commencement of vitamin and iron supplements for the former and placebos for the latter group respectively.

(b) To organise Haemoglobin test of treatment and control group children both before and after administration of drugs as in (a) above.

(c) To keep bi-monthly record of height and weight of the treatment and control group children for purposes of growth monitoring.

(d) To counsel the treatment group mothers about the response action necessary on their part in case of growth-faltering, stagnant weight or weight gain of their respective children.

(e) To administer de-worming treatment to both treatment and control group children before administration of drugs as in (a) above.

(f) To organise a three months long vitamin and iron supplement treatment programme for treatment group children and 'placebos' for the control group as advised by physicians.

(g) To organise referral service for treatment children.

(h) To maintain weekly morbidity data of both treatment and control group children.

(i) To evaluate the impact of health care and growth monitoring inputs on incidence of morbidity data in the treatment group.

(j) To evaluate the impact of health care and growth monitoring inputs on growth of treatment group children as measured by change in their Weight/Height^2 x 100 index.

(k) To evaluate the impact of health care and growth monitoring inputs on the haematological status of the treatment group children.

(l) To evaluate the impact of health and growth-monitoring inputs on the nutritional status of the treatment group children.

1.6.3 *Objectives of the Health Education Programme for the Mothers of Treatment Group children.*

(a) To upgrade knowledge and practice amongst target women regarding:

(i) Ante-natal care.
(ii) Post-natal care.
(iii) Family planning.
(iv) Weaning age and foods.
(v) Balanced diet for children and adults.
(vi) Common nutritive foods with emphasis on those cheaply available.
(vii) Personal hygiene.
(viii) Environmental sanitation.
(ix) Common childhood diseases.
(x) Sickness care and management of the child as specified for each childhood diseases.
(xi) Immunisation—its importance and schedule.
(xii) Existing health services in the neighbourhood and at city level.

(b) To help target women develop more positive attitudes towards:

(i) Health as an asset.
(ii) Female child and women themselves.
(iii) Small family norm.
(iv) Ante-natal care.
(v) Post-natal care.

1.7 Methodology

1.7.1 *Research Design*

The Study undertaken had an experimental design and was conducted in a field setting of Pension-pura slums located in ward number nineteen of Vadodara City.

In a nutshell, it may be stated that the goal of the experiment was to affect measurable improvement in health and growth of slum children under five years through:

(a) Carrying out a package of health care and growth monitoring activities for children themselves.
(b) Imparting a 'situation-practical' health education programme for the mothers of treatment children so as to upgrade latter's knowledge and competence in mothercraft relevant to child health.

Thus there were two independent variables stated as (a) and (b) above and for the sake of convenience denoted as inputs A & B throughout the text. Health of the child was the dependent variable. Operational definitions of all the three variables are given in section 1.7.3.

For evaluation of impact of inputs A & B both Before-After and Treatment-Control (Groups) data were compared and analysed for suitable statistical measures. Before-After comparisons were made to study the impact of planned interventions in the case of same group of children and their respective mothers denoted everywhere as treatment children and treatment mothers.

The experiment also used a matched sample of children and their respective mothers as control groups (Criteria for matching given in section 1.7.6 to make possible an After-only type of comparison between treatment and control groups. This kind of double check was necessary to eliminate any doubts that the treatment groups, over a period of time, might have undergone change attributable to outside influences like mass media or other welfare agencies/workers rather than the interventions by the researcher. (It must be noted that as both treatment and control group children were drawn from the same compact geographical area, outside influences remained a common factor).

1.7.2 *Conceptual Definitions of Independent and Dependent Variables*

Growth-monitoring

Growth is a key indicator of child health. An interplay of ignorance, inappropriate feeding practices, inadequate diet and infection result in one third to half of the children remaining undernourished in the developing world. Malnutrition is a key determinant of the high childhood mortality.

Growth monitoring is advocated and used as a pivotal activity to maintain children on the path of normal growth and development and to recognise early growth faltering. It has been appropriately defined by Bhan M.K. and Ghosh S. (1986:11) as :

> A process of sequential measurement for the assessment of physical growth and development of individual and the community with the purpose of promoting child health, human development and quality of life.

The process involves regular weighing for early identification of growth faltering with appropriate and prompt follow up action. The ultimate target is to educate and achieve change in mother's behaviour towards normal growth and development of the child. The major focus is on child feeding and appropriate response to illness. Growth monitoring provides an excellent opportunity to provide other primary health care services, to improve women's participation and status and interaction between mothers and workers in a predictable and frequent manner.

In fact, growth monitoring activities when properly planned and implemented have a tremendous potential. It, according to World Federation of Public Health Associations (1985:8):

(a) helps identify children with high morbidity/mortality risk;
(b) helps identify parts of the community or the country for special health nutrition;
(c) helps maximise scarce resources for those most in need;
(d) assists in evaluating the impact of the other health intervention activities on the beneficiaries;
(e) does not require a lot of time or expense;
(f) can be carried out realiably by health workers trained at a low cost;
(g) can be organised and run by communities themselves;
(h) offers mothers useful information that, when explained in a culturally relevant manner, provides a basis for understanding and implementing specific dietary improvements;
(i) is a health care activity that can and should be performed without trauma to mother or child;
(j) stimulates collaborative involvement of the health system of the community and the family; and
(k) assumes better preventive and therefore, more effective care for all children.

Growth monitoring is being used in several countries for the past decades or so. In India, it is used on the largest scale in the Integrated Child Development Services (ICDS) programme which has been in operation for more than ten years covering over one fifth of the administrative blocks and approximately 130 million population.

Health

Like the proverbial five blind men who described an elephant each according to his perception, health has been viewed by different people (e.g. biomedical scientists, ecologists, sociologists, anthropologists) from different angles. But for the present purpose definition by World Health Organisation (WHO) has been used as frame of reference. The definition and it is concomitant discussion are as follows:

Health is a state of complete physical, mental and social well-being and not merely an absence of disease or infirmity.

This definition of health envisages three dimensions—Physical, mental and social well-being. According to Twaddle A.C and Hessler R.M (1977) the state of positive health implies the notion of "perfect functioning of the body and mind". It conceptualises health biologically as a state in which every cell and every organ is functioning at optimum capacity and in perfect harmony with the rest of body; psychologically as a state in which the individual feels a sense of perfect well being and of mastery over his environment, and socially, as a state in which the individual's capacities for participation in the social system åre optimal.

The WHO definition is criticised for three major reasons. Firstly, because it does not appear to be a realistic definition of health but is only as idealistic goal which is irrelevent to every day demands and nobody then qualifies as healthy i.e. having perfect biological, psychological and social functioning.

Secondly, some argue that health cannot be defined as a process of continuous adjustment to the changing demands of living and of the changing meanings that we give to life itself.

Thirdly, Crew F.A.W. (1965) contends that this definition does not present health in exact measurable terms.

Despite all these limitations, the concept of health, as defined by WHO is broad and positive in its implications; it sets out the standard—the standard of positive health as a GOAL or IDEAL towards which the people should strive.

Health Education

Health education has been perceived differently by different professionals depending on the specific intents and purposes of the latter. For the present study one of the early definitions by Wilson (1948) has been used. It describes the concept in explicit terms as the process of providing learning experiences for the purpose of influencing knowledge, attitudes and conduct relating to individual, community or World health. It helps individuals to understand how they function as living and dynamic human beings. It makes them alert to understand and appreciate the many factors, obvious as well as subtle which influence health. It acquaints them with community resources for protecting and improving health. It helps them to solve health problems. In short, health education is a modern means to securing widespread understanding and utilisation of present day knowledge concerning health maintenance, improvement and disease prevention. Defined in terms of end results:

> Health education is sum of experiences which favourably influence practices, attitudes and knowledge related to health.

1.7.3 *Operational Definitions of Independent and Dependent Variables*

Independent Variable A

Denotes a package of all health care and growth monitoring interventions for children spread over a span of six months. The package includes:

Organising a thorough medical examination including haemoglobin testing of treatment and control children before administration of prescribed drugs in each group; deworming treatment to both groups; monitoring three month long prescribed treatment for each group; growth-monitoring in case of treatment children only; referral health services to treatment children only; maintaining a weekly morbidity record of both groups throughout six months of interventions; organising after-treatment haemoglobin testing for both groups of children.

Independent Variable B

Refers to a situation practical health education programme for treatment mothers only. The programme comprising of fifteen sessions spread over a period of three months were essentially varied exercises in Group Work practice with the broad aim of enhancing overall competence of target women regarding child health care with added emphasis on underfives. Simplified health messages were communicated through discussions, games, flip chart stories, posters, filmshow, demonstration of nutritive foods, preparation of ORS (Oral Rehydration Salts) mixture and two child-to-child programmes.

Dependent Variable-Health of the Child

For the purposes of present study the dependent variable was operationalised as positive change in Weight/Height^2 x 100 index of growth; haemotological status; and nutritional status as depicted on Road-to-Health cards and a reduction in incidence of morbidity.

1.7.4 *Hypotheses*

At the end of the interventional process the following outcomes were targeted:

Hypothesis one: the mean value of Weight/Height^2 x 100 index of growth in treatment group children would show increase after the experiment vis-a-vis the mean value before. *Two:* the mean value of Weight/height^2 x 100 index of growth in treatment group children vis-a-vis the control group would be higher after the experiment. *Three:* the mean value of haemoglobin level for treatment group children would show increase after the experiment vis-a-vis the mean value before. *Four:* the mean value of haemoglobin level for treatment group children vis-a-vis the control group would be higher after the experiment. *Five:* the mean value of nutritional status for treatment group children would show increase after the experiment vis-a-vis the mean value before. *Six:* the mean value of nutritional status for treatment group children vis-a-vis the control group would be higher after the experiment. *Seven:* the mean reported incidence of each of the eight morbidity conditions viz— diarrhoea, vomitting, measles, chicken pox, skin diseases, high grade fevers, coughs and colds under observation during the intervention period in treatment group would be lower than the corresponding values for control group at the end of the experiment. *Eight:* the mean scores of knowledge (in each unit) pertaining to health care of underfives amongst treatment group mothers would show increase after the health education programme vis-a-vis the corresponding values before. *Nine:* the mean scores of knowledge (in each unit) pertaining to health care of underfives amongst treatment group mothers would be higher than scores obtained by control group after health education programme. *Ten:* the mean scores of attitudes (in each unit) pertaining to health care of underfives amongst treatment group mothers would be higher than control group mothers' score after the health education programme. *Eleven:* the mean scores after the attitudes (in each unit) pertaining to health care of underfives amongst treatment group mothers would be higher than control group mothers' score after the health education programme. *Twelve:* the mean scores of practice (in each unit) pertaining to health care of underfives amongst treatment group mothers' would show increase after the health education programme vis-a-vis the corresponding value before. Thirteen: the mean scores of practice (in each unit) pertaining to health care of underfives amongst treatment group mothers would be higher than the scores obtained by control group mothers after the health education programme.

1.7.5 *Sampling*

The present study being a field experiment, sampling had to be done with much care. Unlike a laboratory, an open community setting does not lend itself to controlled conditions, so vital for any research. The next best course of action we thought, was to locate such slum families which at the time of our planned interventions were not receiving any organised health services at their door step. This could ensure that extraneous influences were kept to a minimum.

First Stage of Sampling

Thus based on the above criteria we selected Harijanvas and Sardargram pockets of Pensionpura slums in Vadodara city where the children were neither covered under the Integrated Child Development Scheme (ICDS) nor by the community service of Childrens' Hospitals, Karelibaug and the like. It was also known that, approximately both the slum pockets together had more than hundred families and there would be a sufficient number of children for study purposes.

Second Stage of Sampling

A base-line survey of Harijanvas and Sadargram families was undertaken to identify the target families, inter alia.

The main criteria for selection of target families was that the family should have atleast one child below 51 months of age of the time of survey, so that the child did not cross the age limit of 5 years before completion of the interventive plan. The second important criterion was willingness of the family, particularly the mother, to participate in the research project.

As such, of the 115 families surveyed, there were 44 families having one or more children less than 51 months of age; the number of these children being 70. Hence the 70 children so identified and their mothers, 44 in number comprised the universe of this study.

The number of children and their mothers were just adequate for study purposes and therefore it was decided to work with all i.e. carry out a census study. Indeed, it must be mentioned here that there were some drop out cases at various stages of intervention period. The miscellaneous reasons being sickness of the child in the first round of clinical investigations, non-cooperation from mothers, temporary absence or permanent move of the family from Pensiónpura etc.

As such, of the 70 eligible children, only 55 received complete package of interventions from the beginning to end; and our data analysis is based on them. Drop out rate thus calculated was 21.4 per cent.

1.7.6 *Criteria for Delineation of Treatment and Control Groups*

Even though the purpose of using matched samples was clear enough *i.e.*, minimising differences due to extraneous variables, the mode of selection of crucial variables required much deliberation. After several permutations and combinations we settled for the following two:

(i) Health Indicator Criteria — Either groups i.e., treatment and control should have equal number of children having haemoglobin levels above 9.0 gms/dl as well as equal numbers having haemoglobin levels below 9.0 gms/dl.

(ii) Socio-economic Indicator Criterion — Either groups *i.e.*, Treatment and control, should have equal number of children having PCI (per capita income) of more than rupees 100 per month as well as an equal number having PCI of less than rupees 100 per month.

Therefore, it was only after the first round of clinical examination *i.e.*, when we had done assessment of haemoglobin levels that the sample was further sub-divided into treatment and control groups. Hence we started with 32 children in the treatment and 30 in the control groups but were left with 30 and 25 respectively in both by the end of intervention as explained earlier in section 1.7.5.

As for the health education programme mothers of the treatment group children were delineated as treatment group mothers while the mothers of the control group children comprised the control group of mothers.

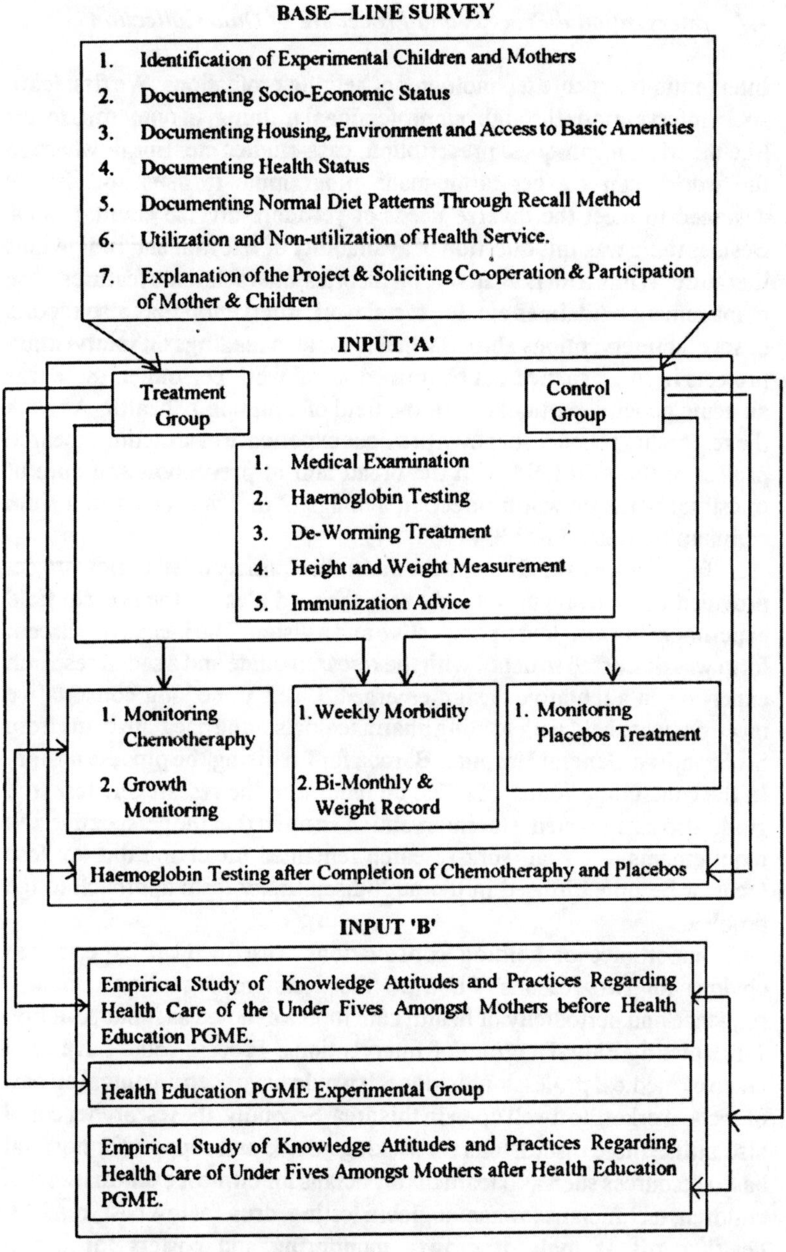

Fig. 1.1: Flow Diagram of Intervention process Base-Line Survey

1.7.7 Interventional Process and Procedure of Data Collection

Interventions are core technologies of helping professions. We first learn about interventions through our professional training, in numerous forms like theories, techniques, prescription, case-studies etc. But nowhere in the world, can we get tailor-made programme formats specifically designed to meet the diverse needs of yet more diverse client groups. Besides there was this question of availability of relevant and indigenous literature. While a lot is available on theories, characteristic features, case management guidelines etc. for social work intervention; as also reports of several interventions abroad when it came to readings on intervention projects in India carried out by trained social work personnel, there was an acute paucity, particularly in the field of community health. As such the researcher relied on her own previous experience of an action research project in the said field with the broad aim of prevention and cure of intestinal parasitic worm infection amongst 3 to 9 years olds in a slum community. Refer Joshi S. (1986: 44).

Experience gained during the multi-disciplinary intervention project provided the researcher not only with the seed idea for the present field experiment but also lent a perspective and a vision. The idea in its nascent form was discussed in detail with the research guide and a social research expert when a tentative design emerged. Later, three joint consultative meetings were held with leading pharmacologists and paediatricians from Sir Sayajirao General Hospital, Baroda for finalising the process design. In the concluding round of talks, on request of the researcher, research guide also participated. Her intervention ensured that the perspective and requirements or social work research remained intact and did not lose focus or become diffused in the multidisciplinary team approach to the problem.

Importance of holding consultations with medical experts was obvious for two reasons. First, all the decisions regarding contents, sequence and periodicity of health care inputs denoted as input A in Fig. 1.1 depicting Flow-Diagram of Interventional Process could have been taken by medical professionals alone. It would have been unethical on part of social workers to dwell upon in this area. Secondly, the researcher could also utilise these discussions for seeking advice and support for hospital based resources such as a team of physicians for clinical examinations of children, technicians for haemoglobin testing, drugs at low cost, road-to-health cards as tools of growth monitoring and posters for health education programme for mothers. Thus an outline of plan of action and tentative calender of intervention tasks was drawn up.

The actual interventional process as shown diagrammatically in Fig. 1.1 had following component blocks:

Base-line survey
Application of Input - A
Application of Input - B

While Fig. 1.1 visually displays key interventive actions under each block and sequence of their occurrence, the procedures used in their implementation and data collection for the study are described here after.

Procedure of Base-line Survey

The researcher first visited the site along with her field work students and met the community men leaders, Mahila Mandal office bearers and some residents to broadly explain the objectives, kind of interventions, expected outcomes etc. and invited their views. It needs to be mentioned here that the researcher has been working through her field work students in this community since July 1981 and a working rapport between us existed before hand. Almost all the persons contacted evinced their interest and inclination to co-operate. On being asked what time would suit them for our door-to-door interviews, they suggested afternoons and also that we could begin any day.

Simultaneously, a semi-structured interview schedule was prepared by the researcher and pilot testing soon began.

The researcher took two students alongwith her each time for demonstration of interview technique and conducted ten interviews over three days. The experience was discussed in group conference for necessary modifications of the schedules as well as mode of interviewing.

The tool was revised as per above and data collected with the help of five field work students placed under researcher at that time. Both pockets were covered within a period of four weeks from 7 Jan '87 to 3 Feb '87. Each respondent was given a token gift of a fibre glass cup which was also used as a measure of consumption of grains and flour per day, thus ensuring fair levels of accuracy and uniformly in data gathered.

Of the 115 families surveyed, 44 families were identified as target families i.e., a family which had at least one child under four years and three months of age (as the child should not cross the age of 5 years before intervention could be duly completed) at the time of interviewing. Immediately, within a week's time analysis of variables like family size, per capita income and any other special health or social condition (like

TABLE: 1.1 Time Schedule of Execution of Component Tasks under Input - A

	Component Task	Time Period
(i)	Organising logistics support	I week Feb '87
(ii)	Pre-interventive haemoglobin test	10 Feb '87
(iii)	Pre-interventive medical examination	19 Feb '87
(iv)	De-worming treatment	IV week Feb '87
(v)	Selection of community health volunteer	"
(vi)	Classification of children into treatment and control groups.	"
(vii)	Bi-monthly height and weight records	Feb, Apr, Jun, Aug '87.
(viii)	Organising and monitoring vitamin and Iron supplements for Treatment children	Apr, May, Jun '87
(ix)	Organising and monitoring placebo treatment for control children	"
(x)	Growth monitoring for treatment children only	Periodically from Feb to Aug '87
(xi)	Weekly record of morbidity amongst Treatment and control groups	Mar to Aug '87
(xii)	Post-intervention haemoglobin testing of treatment and control groups.	30 Aug '87

widowed mother, acute poverty etc.) was completed for the target families.

Later, per capita monthly income and haemoglobin level of the child were used as the two parameters for classifying the experimental children into treatment or control groups (details given earlier).

Procedures in Application of Input A

Despite the long drawn strike by junior government doctors at Baroda in early 1987, we got full logistics support from SSG Hospitals for various clinical examinations and were able to work as per the tentative plan of action.

We on our part also made detailed and systematic advance preparations to secure optimum success in each task undertaken and corresponding data collection. Such preparations included prior intimation to community women about the forthcoming events; on-the-spot persuasion in case of some women for haemoglobin test of their children or giving vitamin and iron supplement pills/syrup to the child without fail; preparation of forms for record of medical examination with the help of doctors; issuing registration cards to each child to facilitate co-ordination of various tests; advance preparation of registers for record of haemoglobin level, height, weight, recommended treatment, referrals if any, and weekly morbidity data; training and monitoring role of community health volunteer; explaining road-to-health cards to mothers etc.

The people's support was evident by their arranging of tables, chairs and test equipments; maintaining order on the spot as there used to be more than 50 children and their mothers each time with many children screaming loudly because of blood test or fear of it; offering water and tea to the clinical team and social workers present etc.

Table 1.1 above on p. 34 depicts time schedule of all component tasks under input A

Procedure in Application of Input 'B'

As shown in Fig. 1.1 input B comprised of three major tasks, namely:

(a) Empirical study of Knowledge, Attitudes and Practices (KAP) regarding healthcare of underfives amongst mothers of both treatment and control groups before health education programme conducted for treatment group only.
(b) Construction and implementation of a situation practical health education programme (HEP) for mothers of treatment group only.
(c) Empirical study of KAP regarding health care of underfives amongst mothers of both treatment and control groups after health education programme conducted for treatment group only.

A semi-structured and pre-coded KAP measurement scale covering all the areas of inquiry mentioned under the objectives of HEP was developed after a careful scrutiny of related literature and discussion with experts from medical and social science professions. The scale after proper pre-testing and necessary modifications was administered on mothers of both treatment and control groups; and thus pre-intervention data was collected.

Next came the actual implementation of HEP consisting of fifteen sessions spread over a period of three months approximately from Jul 24, '87 to Oct 31, '87. The sessions were held at the 'Balwadi' in Sardargram usually in the afternoon as per the convenience of the participants.

In the very first session, the participants were oriented about the goals, subject content, programme duration and teaching methods to be used during the HEP. Next, the working modalities with regard to timings, duration and periodicity of the sessions, incentives for high attendance and merit performance etc. were discussed with the participants. Decisions were taken on the basis of majority vote. The same session included three short educational games. In the end, the women were informed that Fatehganj Samaj Kalyan Kendra, an extension agency of Faculty of Social Work, M.S. University would award them certificates subject to successful completion of the course by the participants.

Of the remaining fourteen sessions, the last one was reserved for Certificates Award and Prize Distribution Function. For each of the preceding thirteen sessions, objectives, media of instruction and audio-visual aids were carefully planned in advance. Preparations for the sessions in terms of developing an aid, contacting resource person for talks, training the children for a skit or rally was done separately in additional hours which at times extended over one or two weeks as in the case of the latter two items just mentioned.

Coming to the subject matter content, we were aware that some areas were rather 'difficult' for the participants (to comprehend) as they had never heard of these or practiced them before *e.g.* a balanced meal, role and functions of different nutrients, information on certain childhood diseases etc. Under the circumstances, in order to sustain the interest and involvement of the participants throughout the intervention period we deployed a whole gamut of communication techniques, namely—group discussion, talks aided by charts and posters, talks by outside experts, paper presentation by volunteers from the learners' group, educative games, story telling, health quiz, skit, rally, cooking demonstration and film show.

In short, it may be said that the present HEP model was an exercise in Group Work practice with sharply defined goals; the setting being an urban slum community.

Post intervention data was collected on the same scale by different investigations; again for both treatment and control group mothers.

1.7.8 *Reliability and Validity of KAP Scale*

Reliability means repeatability of the measuring instrument or the level of consistency in the answers obtained by it. As earlier mentioned, for the present study, no ready-made commercial scale with a given reliability value was available. We, therefore, not only had to develop a KAP scale of our own but also had to ascertain its reliability. Test-Retest method was used.

Ten mothers out of the thirty which comprised the experimental group *i.e.*, 33.3 per cent were interviewed a second time by a different

TABLE: 1.2 Reliability Test of KAP Scale

Sl. No.	Sub-Scale Item	R-Value
1.	Knowledge of Diarrhoea	.75544
2.	Knowledge of Measles	.95343
3.	Knowledge of Chicken Pox	.83923
4.	Knowledge of Anaemia	.97225
5.	Knowledge of Tetanus	.86621
6.	Knowledge of Scabies	.53157
7.	Knowledge of Infant feeding	.87830
8.	Knowledge of Nutritious Diet	.97488
9.	Knowledge of Pre-natal care	.61496
10.	Knowledge of Post-natal care	.67900
11.	Knowledge of Family Planning	.98939
12.	Knowledge of Immunization schedule and advantages	.82151
13.	Knowledge of Health services in neighbourhood and at city level.	.66310
14.	Attitude to Infant Feeding	.92125
15.	Attitude to Family Planning	.97646
16.	Attitude towards women and Female Children	.76771
17.	Attitude towards health professionals and Services	.68552
18.	Practice of infant feeding	.93276
19.	Practice of Sickness care of child	.88024
20.	Practice of personal Hygiene	.96104

investigator within five weeks of the first interview. The scale itself consisted of twenty sub-scales each of which was complete by itself. Hence the scores obtained by the individual respondents in the first and second round of inquiry were analysed for their correlation matrix, and the R-value was calculated by Cronbach's Alpha formula. The results are presented in Table 1.2.

Table 1.2 shows that the R-value of various sub-scale items ranged between a minimum of .53157 as for knowledge of scabies to maximum of .98939 as in the case of 'knowledge of Family Planning'. Thirteen out of twenty sub-scale items had an R-value of more than .80 which is considered high enough for standardizing and commercialising of a scale. Two other items, namely, 'knowledge of Diarrhoea' and 'Attitude towards Women and Female Children' had R-value above .75 and it can be said that it was good enough. The remaining five items had low R-value of less than .70.

In order that the KAP scale was high on validity *i.e.* it indeed measured what it was purported to have measured; the questions contained by the scale were drafted very carefully with reference to a theoretical frame work excerpted from Training Manual on Research Methodology on Child Labour and Health (1984: 37) as per below:

Responses to questions are less likely to be valid at least in three circumstances:

(1) If the questions are embarrassing, such as those involving sexual functions or bowel habits;
(2) If honest responses might endanger the subject (for example, a child might suffer physical punishment or loss of his job if he tells an interviewer that his employer is abusive).
(3) If there is a motive to gain some social effect, such as to amuse the interviewer, or gain his respect or approval. Children especially are likely to guess at what answers might please an adult.
(4) Some times respondents will give answers even when they don't understand the question, either to please the interviewer or just to get the interview over with.

Further since internal validity of a classical experimental design such as the one used in the present study is characteristically strong as per Powers G.T. *et al.* (1985: 206), it was felt that additional validity of the measurement scale was not really necessary. Here, the classical experimental design would essentially have four characteristics as follows:

First, there is a manipulated independent variable. In a TRUE experiment, the causal variable or the independent variable is administered or changed by the experimenter in order to ensure the time order.

Second, is the existence of at least one dependent variable.

Third, common feature of true experiments is the random assignment of subjects to experimental and control groups. This equalizes the groups when the experiment begins.

The Fourth, trait of the experimental design is the process of pre-testing and post-testing.

1.7.9 *Data Analysis and Presentation*

With reference to the objectives of the study, voluminous data was collected which for purpose of organised presentation can be placed in three broad categories as shown below:

(i) Base-line survey data;
(ii) Data pertaining to health and growth monitoring (of children) interventions; and
(iii) Data pertaining to health education interventions (programme for mothers).

While, the base-line data was analysed by the researcher with the aid of a scientific calculator, the other categories (ii) & (iii) stated above were computer processed at EDP section of Tata Institute of Social Sciences, Bombay. For the latter categories ICSSR research grant for guidance and consultancy services in statistics and Electronic Data Processing was utilised.

Chapter three presents findings of the base line survey which essentially highlight socio-economic profiles of the sample besides some related statistics on the health of underfives in the community. Frequency and percentage distribution; means and standard deviation: and mode are the statistical measures used herein.

Discussion of impact of social interventions on health and growth of study children is presented in chapter four. Student's t-test was applied to verify relevant hypotheses from one to seven. Multiple regression analysis was used to study the effect of independent variables like household size, mother's age, mother's education and per capita monthly income on the indexed dependent variables like weight/height^2 x 100; haemoglobin status and nutritional status.

Chapter five presents analysis of impact of health education programme conducted for treatment mothers. As in earlier chapter four, Student's t-test was applied to verify the relevant hypothesis from eight to thirteen and multiple regression analysis was used to study the effect of independent variables like household size, mother's age, per capita monthly income and mother's education on dependent variables like change in aggregate scores of knowledge, attitude and practice of target mothers.

1.7.10 *Need, Selection and Role of Community Health Volunteer*

Health and growth surveillance of 55 children involving a broad range of interventions over a period of six months as the cornerstone of the present study demanded a live day-to-day contact with the field and target people. In search of a suitable device fulfilling the above requirements, we decided to keep the trusted counsel of reaching the community through a local, well-liked, responsible, resident volunteer. The researcher having known Pensionpura people for some years had three suitable women candidates in mind and had been seeking students' opinion regarding who would suit the role best when the selection issue clinched itself on the first day of the clinical examination. K (one of the three candidates) doing a marvellous job of helping the medical and social workers team on her own drew everybody's attention. It was a good demonstration of a situation throwing up leadership potential from the community. All of us present there felt that the part time post of CHV should be first offered to K. Only in case she declined it, should we approach others. Besides, her quiet leadership abilities, K was literate and in the past had done a meticulous job of account keeping as the treasurer of Sardargram Mahila Mandal. Soon the offer was made to her alongwith the explanation of what was expected of her. We were indeed happy when she readily agreed to join us.

Following tasks were assigned to the CHV:

(a) Visit target families every Tuesday to inquire about the health of study children and report to the researcher the following day with the morbidity data register. In case of emergencies, she was to report immediately anytime during the week;

(b) To help field work students in extending follow up or referral service to the ailing child;

(c) To guide treatment group mothers in completing immunisation of their children from time to time as advised by the researcher;

(d) To distribute vitamins, iron supplements and 'placebos' to children as advised by the researcher;

(e) To help researcher in collecting height and weight of all children once in two months; and

(f) To help researcher and students during health education sessions by taking care of small children accompanying their mothers.

The necessary training for the above listed tasks was personally given by the researcher through demonstration & discussions with the CHV.

In a summary evaluative comment on the performance of CHV it may be said that she not only did a commendable job but that her own personality also showed growth as the project progressed.

1.8 Limitations of the Study

First and foremost, the limitations built into our conceptual frame work itself.

To begin with, let us scrutinise the issue of delineating several children with very poor general health (as indicated by their low haemoglobin levels) into control group of the study design; thus receiving only 'placebos' for three months. Was it so essential to have matched samples for treatment and control groups? Was it not feasible to select some criterion other than haemoglobin status for sampling purpose? We debated at length over the above posers amongst ourselves as well as with the medical consultants. And obviously, having failed to come up with a superior alternative reconciled to compromise our humanitarian concern for sake of an un-ambiguous research model.

Secondly, research scientists can always argue (and quite justifiably) that the sample size for study of impact of health education programme was too small. There were only 13 (though we started with 15, there were 2 drop-outs) and 15 mothers in treatment and control groups respectively and one can always question the worth of generalisations based on t-test results for both independent and paired samples. The extenuating circumstance was however this that the decision on the sample size of mothers' group in a sense, was not left to us. The total number of both groups was 30 and they were the mothers of 55 children who were our main research clients under the study. Several mothers were having two children under 51 months of age but got included in the sample size only once. The relatively low mean age of the mothers *i.e.* 25.441 years with the standard deviation of the sample as 3.895 years clarifies further how it came to be that many mothers had two or occasionally three children below 5 years.

Lastly, paucity of earlier experimental research in this field particularly on Indian soil, was a real handicap.

2

SOCIAL INTERVENTION
Some Core Precepts And Field Projects

In order to ensure optimum impact of the experimental research work reported here, an exhaustive study of theoretical issues related to social (work) intervention as well as strategies, techniques and programme format adopted by some field intervention projects in Child Health was undertaken before finalising the methodology. Thus, the voluminous literature reviewed, for the present purposes can be summarised into two major sections as follows:

Section 2.1: covering some theoretical precepts on Social Intervention and its core aspects by established authors on the subject; and

Section 2.2: Presenting an overview of actual intervention projects and research studies on growth-monitoring and health of underfives in India.

It may be pinpointed here at the very outset that all the studies in this area came mainly from two allied disciplines of nutrition and medicine while quite ironically, only a little was available from professional social work.

SECTION 2.1

REVIEWS: SOME THEORETICAL PRECEPTS ON SOCIAL INTERVENTION

An exhaustive review of literature on the subject presents a high level of concurrence amongst leading social scientists on the concept of intervention. Few definitions by established authors substantiate the above observation. According to Algyris C. (1970: 15) to intervene is to enter into an ongoing system of relationship, to come between or among persons or objects for the purpose of helping them. There is an important implicit assumption in the definition that should be made explicit: the system exists independently of the intervenor. Thomas (1984: 29) stipulated the element of planning in intervention as per his definition; intervention is a planned intrusion into the life or environment of an individual, couple, family or other target unit that is intended to bring about beneficial changes for the individual or others involved. Compton and Galaway (1984: 11) highlight active participation by the client in the intervention process when according to them—intervention refers to deliberate, planned actions by the client and worker to resolve a problem. Thus intervention occurs after a problem has been defined and after the desired resolution (or the goal) has been identified. In practice, when interventions are accompanied by research objectives it becomes necessary to distinguish between intervention research and action research. Fineman (1985: 15) differentiating between the two, says that unlike much action research, the end of intervention research is not just client action or change: the researcher has his or her own particular conceptual interests. The intervention provides a vehicle for exploring these interests, perhaps describing a situation, generating new concepts, or testing some hunches or hypotheses.

2.1.1 *Social Work and Social Intervention*

Primary concern of social work profession being people-in-their-life-situations where they have to constantly strike a delicate balance between compulsions of their social environment on one hand and their capacity to cope with on the other; Zastrow (1990) had defined social work principles, skills, techniques and values for helping individuals; groups, or communities to enhance or restore their capacity for psycho-social functioning and to create societal conditions favourable to their goals. The professional values and the scientific body of knowledge equip the practitioner with the right skills and attitudes towards people in their situation and facilitate his/her helping role while working independently or in collaborative action.

Social work intervention is often discharged through use of a single method or a combination of methods as found necessary. Following are the six widely recognized methods of social work profession:

(i) *Social Case Work* is aimed at helping individuals, on a one-to-one basis, to enhance or restore their psycho-social functioning through application of professional principles, skills, techniques and values;

(ii) *Group Work* is a process of social work in which the qualified worker helps individuals in a group by providing a desirable group experience through various programme media with a view to enabling members to move towards improved social relationships and their psycho-social functioning.

(iii) *Community Organisation* is the process of stimulating and assisting the local community to identify, evaluate, plan and co-ordinate its efforts to meet its own "felt" and "un-felt" needs and develop cooperative and collaborative spirit in working together.

(iv) *Social Work Administration* involves directing the overall programme of a social service agency. Administrative functions include setting agency and programme objectives, analyzing social conditions in the community and making decisions about what services will be provided, employing and supervising staff members, setting up an organizational structure administering financial affairs and securing funds for the agency's operations.

(v) *Social Action* is concerned with changing the social environment to meet the recognized needs of individuals or disadvantaged groups by application of tactics involving conflict, confrontation and negotiations.

(vi) *Social Work Research* may be defined as systematic investigation intended to add to available knowledge in a form that is communicable and verifiable.

Social Work Research is applied research which aims to contribute to the development of a dependable body of knowledge to serve the goals and means of social work in all its remifications.

2.1.2 *Pre-conditions for Intervention Activity*

Are there any basic or necessary conditions that must be fulfilled, if intervention activity is to be impactful?

One condition that seems so basic as to be considered axiomatic is the generation of valid information. Without valid information, it would be difficult for the client to learn and for the interventionist to help.

A second condition almost as basic is that interventions should be so designed and executed that the client system maintains its discreteness and autonomy. Thus, free, informed choice is also a necessary process in an effective intervention activity.

Finally, if the client system is ongoing (existing over time), the clients require strengthening to maintain their autonomy not only vis-a-vis the interventionist but also vis-a-vis other systems. This means that their commitment to learning and change has to be more than temporary. It has to be so strong that it can be transferred to relationships other than those of the interventionist and can do so (eventually) without the help of the latter. The third basic process for any intervention activity is, therefore the client's internal commitment to the choice made.

2.1.3 *Levels of Intervention*

There are three levels of intervention, *viz.*, primary prevention, crisis intervention and secondary intervention. More about each level follows.

Primary Prevention—This involves anticipating and forestalling the eruption of conflict, in an individual, family or community, especially that which could result in some sort of setback or violence. For instance, research indicates that the period around birth offers a unique opportunity for assessing parents and their babies for potential problems in their interaction with each other—Gray *et al.* (1976); Schneider *et al.* (1976)' and Dean *et al.* (1987). Similarly, if we could identify violence prone couples at an early stage in their relationships, should we place them on At Risk Registers and what kind of supportive intervention be introduced? Supportive action could range from introducing more effective educational programmes to help people anticipate common problems in family life to counselling certain couples not to live together or get married—The Open University (1980). In our local setting illustrations of Juvenile Guidance Centres or School Readiness Programmes can be given as interventions for Primary Prevention.

Crisis intervention—This may involve rescuing the victim or removing the perpetrator of abuse and further help restore some measure of equilibrium immediately after a crisis, providing relief from conflict on a temporary basis, or using a crisis for long term ends. The term is frequently misunderstood and misused especially in relation to situations of conflict and violence. For example, it is used indiscriminately to describe both family's crisis and the professional's or community's anxious response often in form of piecemeal, adhoc intervention. It must be noted that, crisis theory is about the family's or community's accessibility to change and not about the level of anxiety or urgency in the professionals or the community. Inter alia, crisis intervention theory suggests that during crisis often individual's or family's usual methods of coping with problems prove inadequate and events which in themselves may seem trivial or unimportant become linked with earlier experiences and therefore trigger off unresolved or partly resolved conflicts from the past. By definition, the period of crisis does not last long and within a few weeks a new equilibrium is usually reached according to the kind of help received and the individual's or families' adaptive capacities.

In Indian setting, cases of pregnancy out of wedlock, rape, sudden deformity or disabilities resulting from accidents or illnesses, failure in love or board examinations, death of a close relative or friend, natural or manmade disasters etc. could precipitate genuine crisis needing crisis intervention.

Secondary Intervention—This may be short-term or long-term intervention. It involves superficial monitoring of a situation to contain recurrence of violence or destruction and any further deteriorating trends. In this context, it may include affecting fundamental changes in individuals or whole families, their personality, behaviour, patterns of interaction or environmental and social circumstances. To accomplish the aforesaid intervention goals any of the following techniques, alone or in a judicious combination may be used; case work; psychotherapy; psychoanalysis—in few cases; positive reinforcement; direct provision of material aid; affecting major or minor structural change in local community or society through social action; recourse to legal aid; teaching of social and communication skills; mobilizing resources for creation of services like housing, recreation, day care centres for young, elderly, handicapped or any other vulnerable group: catalysing formation of self help groups like tenants' association, alcoholics' anonymous; Dalit Kranti Sangh (Organisation of the downtrodden); Wali Mandal (Parents' Association) etc.

2.1.4 *Dimensions of Intervention*

Conceptual clarity of various dimensions of intervention considerably help in selection of specific intervention approaches. These dimensions as highlighted by The Open University (1980: 25) are:

1. how causal factors are perceived and identified;
2. with relation to the aims and desired outcomes, whether the emphasis and level of intervention is on prevention, on dealing with and utilizing crisis, on control and maintenance or on

implementing change (e.g. by promoting growth, or relieving symptoms or problems);
3. whether the focus is on an individual, two people, an entire family or a wider network;
4. whether the emphasis is on the past or the present, on experience or behaviour, on utilizing apparent strengths or focusing on pathology;
5. whether the emphasis is on offering professional help and support or an encouraging self help; and
6. whether statutory authority and responsibility exist;
7. how much time, knowledge, skill and other resources are available to those who intervene.

2.1.5 *Objectives of Intervention or Change Objectives*

Change objectives indicate the goals towards which the efforts of helping should be directed and can influence all components of the helping strategy/intervention design. Some of the principle objectives relevant to intervention design alongwith their brief description and relevant examples are summarized in Table 2.1

While each objective with its own strengths and limitations has a legitimate place in social intervention, the objective of remediation is the most common and widespread problems calling for remediation are generally quite pressing and intervention methods directed towards remediation have been the best developed. More about each objective may be read from, Table 2.1 Contemporary intervention has often been criticized because it does not focus sufficiently on the vital objectives of competence and prevention. However, fortunately of late, attitudes are changing for the better and interventions focussing on competence and prevention are now beginning to receive the attention they deserve.

2.1.6 *Planning for Intervention*

The purpose of establishing an intervention plan in the first place is to know where we want to go and how we are going to get there. While such a plan does not guarantee that we will reach our destiny, it does improve our chances of getting there and reduces the probability of our getting lost on the way.

All the therapists, therefore, must formulate treatment plans that identify intervention methods appropriate for addressing particular client concerns. The fashioning of an intervention plan calls for consideration

TABLE: 2.1 : Selected Change Objectives with Examples

Change Objective	What It Is	Examples
Remediation	Intervention directed toward altering a problem that is a source of difficulty for the client	Providing assertive training for an unssertive young person. Sex therapy for a young man with psychological impotence, or communication training for marital partners who disagree excessively.
Enhancement	Intervention directed toward improving functioning above an already satisfactory level	Providing a sexual improvement programme for marital partners whose sexual adjustment is already satisfactory to make the sexual satisfaction greater or a parent training programme for parents whose children do not have severe problems and who already handle most problems well.
Competence	Intervention directed toward strengthening the client's ability to handle not only an existing difficulty but also a variety of difficulties in a given area, including those that may rise in that area in the future.	By focusing on self-inducted relaxation and cognitive coping providing anxiety management training for individuals who also have other areas of anxiety, doing so in such a way as to strengthen the individual's ability to manage existing anxieties as well as anxiety-evoking situations that may come up later; training parents to handle any of a variety of child management difficulties that may be presented now and later.
Education	The presentation of information to facilitate understanding in an area of intervention.	Presenting information to the family of a substance abuser concerning for example, the nature of the substance, its adverse effects, the typical course of addiction, possible ways in which the family members may cope with the ill effects of the substance abuse, and how they may assist in rehabilitation.
Prevention	Intervention directed toward eliminating potential difficulties before they arise or become sufficiently problematic to require remediation	Training adolescent children in secondary school in conflict resolution, communication and decision making to provide the participants with skill so that possible future discord in intimate relationships would be averted.

Advocacy	Speaking up for and taking other actions on behalf of the client to protect the client's rights and to pursue client interests.	Assisting the client to take legal action in connection with alleged discrimination; negotiating for the client to obtain more satisfactory housing.
Resource	Provision of such resources as food, clothing, shelter, money or medicine.	Giving food to the unemployed who have exhausted unemployment benefits; providing shelter to flood victims.
Social Control	Interventions directed toward protection of the client and/or society generally through provision of special residential arrangements.	Incarceration of legal offenders establishing separate residential facilities for the mentally impaired, the aged, or those terminally ill.

Excerpted from : *Designing Interventions for the Helping Professions* by Thomas, E.J., Sage Publications, Beverley Hills, 1984 pp. 31.

of suitable alternatives, given available methods, as well as new approaches that might be adopted to meet the problem in question.

Although carried out with a particular client or clients for given service purposes, such planning is a limited form of design that can result in producing a novel intervention for cases of that type. Powers *et al.* (1985: 203) have highlighted the major considerations that need to be made before an intervention plan is drawn up.

Firstly, they point out that in planning strategy for intervention, it is important that the client and practitioner agree on the immediate, intermediate and long range goals to be pursued. Goals not only provide incentive and direction for what is to be achieved, but they also provide an objective basis for determining achievement itself. Further, there should be mutual agreement between the professional and clients on relevant issues like—who will be expected to do what; where is it to take place; within what time frame is it to be accomplished? Such commitments by the involved parties, in turn, provide the basis for what may be thought of as "working contract" or agreement concerning the division of labour.

The above stated are not the only questions that need to be addressed in planning intervention. For example, who or what should be identified as the target of intervention? The fact that the client experiences a problem does not necessarily mean that he or she should be viewed as either having caused it or as having it within his or her power to do anything about it. It is important, therefore, to identify precisely where the locus of change is (to take place)—in the client, or in some other facet of the client's environment? What systems will need to be involved in the change process besides the client—the client's family, his or her work place, the school systems, additional human service agencies, or other community systems or organisations that either directly or indirectly impinge upon the client's life?

Next consideration is of the modes of intervention to be employed in the practitioner's attempt to resolve the situation—work with an individual or family, use a group, organize a resource system in the community, or some combination of two or more of those. Clients like other people, differ widely with respect to motivation and/or capacity to participate in various practice modalities.

It is also important to be clear as to who should be included among the change agents. Practitioners and clients themselves are rarely the ones who can affect change in the client's situation. In fact, in some instances they may be relatively powerless to do so. Therefore, consideration needs to be given to the question of what other resources within the environment might be brought within the purview of the change process.

And finally the important issue of the practitioner's orientation to practice itself. Practitioners differ widely in their perspective—a perspective that influences everything, from the assumptions they make about people and their problems, to the way they define the nature of client-practitioner relationship, and to the selection of the very practice techniques they rely upon to promote change.

2.1.7 *Intervention Methods*

Intervention methods are the backbone of the anatomy of the helping process and are generally central in intervention design. Further the methods are composed of one or more intervention techniques and a program format.

The intervention technique is a recognized and distinctive set of helping activities that relate to a particular interventional objective. Many intervention techniques are largely accelerative or decelerative. The accelerative technique is used to increase desirable responding whereas the decelerative technique is intended to decrease undesirable responding. Providing re-inforcement in the form of praise to a child for doing his or her homework is illustrative of an accelerative technique. On the other hand, reducing pocket money (Say, a day's allowance) for incomplete homework would work as a decelerative technique. Few generalisations about the accelerative and decelerative techniques are as below:

1. All things considered, accelerative techniques are preferred over the decelerative. In the aforesaid example, if Chinky fails to do her homework regularly, it would be more profitable to announce additional pocket allowance for the completion of homework by her rather than reducing the allowance for incomplete work.
2. There are often negative effects of using a decelerative technique—for example, undesirable emotional reactions alongwith associating the therapist and the situation of intervention with unpleasant and aversive consequences.
3. Deceleration need not and often does not bring about a simultaneous increase in the desired responding.
4. Accelerative techniques are not always powerful by themselves. There are difficult situations of behaviour change in which even the strongest and best techniques may be ineffective. In such contexts both accelerative and decelerative techniques can be used in combination. For instance, in addition to earning special pocket allowance for completion of homework Chinky could also lose her hours of TV veiwing for failing to do it (homework).

The above stated dual approach is the preferred alternative in situations in which either type of technique by itself would being uncertain or unsatisfactory results.

Program Format, the second component of an intervention method is the assembly of intervention elements (consisting of one or more intervention techniques). Programmes may vary greatly in format depending on such factors as their scope, number of interventions, order of intervention, strength of intervention, longevity and structure. Brief observations on the aforesaid factors determining the programme format follow:

1. There is increasing recognition that the scope of intervention in a program should include more than the target behaviour itself—for example, the controlling conditions for the behaviour related system and environmental influences. For example, a health education intervention aiming to upgrade mothers' skills in health care of underfive children should also impart knowledge of prevention of common childhood diseases and how to care for the ailing child; information of immunization and other health services available in neighbourhood and at city level; understanding of the concept of a balanced meal etc. as done in the present project.
2. Although the variety of techniques need not always be large to

be effective, there should be a sufficient number of appropriate techniques to accomplish the intervention object. Variety in application of techniques sustains clients' interest and also improves the extent of clients' gains from the programme.

3. The strength of intervention should be neither too weak not too strong; rather it should be sufficiently potent to achieve the intervention objective.
4. When determining the extent to which the programme should be individualized or standardized, attention needs to be given to such factors as the appropriateness of the programme for the individuals involved, the cost in time and effort and programme benefits for clients. For example, it would be highly efficacious to undertake a base-line survey of knowledge, attitudes and practices of health care amongst mothers of underfives in a given community before launching forth a health education intervention program for them (mothers). The gleanings from the base-line study would facilitate the task of designing a program format which is 'situation-practical'.
5. While there are advantages of time-bound interventions, the time allowed for interventions should be certainly enough to carry out the intervention competently.
6. Programs may be structured as tight or loose, each of which has advantages and disadvantages depending on the characteristics of the participant clients, the degree of risk in the event of program non-compliance, and the stage of development of interventions.
7. To increase the likelihood that interventions will yield long-term generalised benefits, ideally interventions should be carefully designed at the very outset. For example, interventions that draw heavily on strengths and resources of clients, of mediators and of conditions prevailing in the environment are more likely to facilitate generalized change than interventions which rely more on professionals and agency personnel.

2.1.8 *Dilemmas of Intervention*

There is a fundamental dilemma of intervention with which all practitioners are confronted sometime or other. This dilemma may be expressed variously as whether the effect of their intervention can be deemed as positive or negative; whether the advantages of their intervention outweigh the disadvantages; and whether, in fact, they are helping or hindering their clients. Inevitably such issues involves value judgements as well as objective measurement. More specifically, as per The Open University Text (1980: 36) consider the following maxims in the context of a family where conflict has resulted in violence:

1. Protecting one family member may mean controlling another.
2. One kind of safety may be achieved at the price of different kind of risk.

While there can be no formatted answers to the poser above, interventionists can certainly fall back on a few tested 'dos' in their work as explained below:

Firstly, it is emphasized that although at times effective protection is vital, practitioners should be careful that protection of those in danger should not take an unduly provocative form as many victims may find themselves back in the same household at a later date. For example, in order to protect a legally minor girl from an impending marriage, the interventionist should not lodge a police complaint against the parents of the client because such action would leave permanent scars on the parent-child relationship even if the undesirable marriage is forestalled. The damaged parent-child relationship could possibly arouse further tension and violence.

Secondly, all practitioners need to be aware that any intervention by outsiders is a family life, even if it is at a seemingly simple level or focussed on only one member of a family, may have a considerable impact on all the immediate family and may have repercussions on their extended family or social network. Indeed, the impact or repercussions could either be positive or negative. For instance, if one spouse has taken recourse to professional marital counselling, the other spouse may or may not view it favourably. Therefore, the practitioner needs to be alert when he or she approaches the other spouse, as part of the intervention plan.

Lastly, decisions about intervention in the lives of adult citizens should be made as far as possible by those citizens themselves. There is always the danger, that practitioners, especially when intervening in a crisis, will get pulled into taking charge of another adult citizen's life because that client presents himself/herself in such a passive or vulnerable way that he does not make decisions which are his to make. This serves as a note of caution to the practitioner before he/she takes drastic actions like rescuing victims by removing them elsewhere, unless of course, they are in acute danger. The practitioner should first explore whether another form of temporary relief or support might be a sufficient safeguard.

Further, an assessment whether the crisis in itself can be used to bring about change and serve long-term ends must be acted upon. And finally, the consideration whether once the current crisis has passed and been dealt with what sort of long-term support is indicated?

2.1.9 *Programme Evaluations*

Programme evaluation as a subject has several dimensions, of which many deserve a detailed study and discussion. However, in this paper we shall highlight three aspects: what is programme evaluation; why do programme evaluation; and various ways to categorize programme evaluation designs.

It is always helpful to begin with definitions. While there are numerous authorities on the subject we quote here Attkisson and Broskowski (1978: 24) for their all inclusive definition according to which—

Programme evaluation involves

1. A process of making reasonable judgements about programme effort, effectiveness, efficiency and adequacy;
2. Based on systematic data collection and analysis.
3. Designed for use in programme management; external accountability and future planning.
4. Focusses especially on accessibility, acceptability, awareness, availability, comprehensiveness, continuity, integration and cost of services.

Coming to the question— "why do programme evaluations"? It seems strange that this question be raised at all. That is because programme evaluations more often than not have been viewed as integral to agency operations for standard reasons. The reasons being:

First, agencies are expected to be accountable to clients, communities and funders for both funds and programme effectiveness. Second, managers need the information generated in evaluation to make decisions about internal operations and programme changes. Third, practitioners use programme evaluation data for assessing client progress, for self-assessment and for their own professional development. Fourth, programme evaluation is good for community relations, for establishing agency creditability.

While there are several ways to categorise programme evaluation designs, we present here a frame work by Rossi P.H. and Freeman H.E. (1982: 33). They discuss four types of evaluation activities:

1. *Programme Planning*—These are research activities designed to describe an agency's target population and its needs and to assess whether a specific programme has been developed and implemented in such a way as to meet its goals.
   This is frequently called "needs assessment" research. It is the most common form of evaluation of a programme in its early stages of development, while initial planning is being done.
2. *Programme monitoring*—These research activities measure whether the agency is delivering the programme as intended and whether the programme's services are reaching the intended target. Administrators find monitoring activities extremely useful in assessing how the programme is operating and whom it serves.
3. *Programme impact*—Evaluation of programme impact measures the amount of change in a desired direction that can be attributed to the programme intervention. It is necessary to use carefully controlled research designs to assess the impact of a programme and be certain the measured impact was caused by the programme. The evaluation of programme impact should be done after the programme has been developed beyond its initial planning stages and when services are being delivered. Impact evaluation is what most people mean when they talk about programme evaluation.
4. *Programme Efficiency*—Activities to assess the programme's economic efficiency include the measurement of the costs and the outcomes or the benefits of the programme. This evaluation builds on the impact evaluation and further assesses whether the programme uses resources efficiently.

Most agencies use one or more of these evaluations in the standard operations of their programmes. A comprehensive approach to evaluation would include a number of them.

SECTION 2.2

CONTAINS ANALYTICAL REVIEW OF ACTUAL INTERVENTION PROJECTS

In this section on discussion of actual intervention projects in the area of growth-monitoring and health of underfives, we first take up voluntary effort by intervention health agencies; then move on to voluntary work of local organisations and finally present the state level efforts, while extracts of relevant research studies would be presented at the end.

2.2.1 The Narangwal Project is the most talked about project in the field of growth monitoring and health of underfives (0-3 years old) in India. The project was carried out by the Department of Interventional health at the John Hopkins University in ten villages in Narangwal, Punjab, India during 1968 and 1973. Accordingly to Kakkar (1987) the following were some of the policy questions which led to the Narangwal Study:

(i) Can nutrition interventions reduce the incidence, duration and impact of infections?
(ii) Can control of infection improve nutritional status?
iii) Is there a synergism in programme effects so that a combined nutrition and infection control programme would have a greater cost-effectiveness than what would be expected from each programme alone?
(iv) Can better field programmes be developed to combine the most effective measures against mal-nutrition and infection so that these measures can be implemented within the existing constraints?

Ten study villages in four clusters of two or three villages each scattered around community development blocks were earmarked for differential child health services. Careful attention was paid to keep the village clusters separate to minimize communications between them about differences in the packages that were offered to them. The service package received by the four clusters differentially were: (1) nutrition care, (2) health care with main emphasis in infection control, (3) integrated services *i.e.*, both nutrition and health care, (4) a control group which received no health service other than emergency aid. All children were under growth surveillance.

Results pertaining to Growth and Development

(i) Nutrition care alone or in combination with health care significantly improved both weight and height of children studied beyond 17 months of age;
(ii) At 36 months, children from the nutrition care villages weighed on an average 560 gms. more and were 1.3 cm. taller than children in the control villages;
(iii) Children in the health care villages had mean weights and

heights intermediate between those in the nutrition care and control villages; and

(iv) Of the socio-economic and demographic variables, sex and caste were shown to have an especially pronounced and additive effect.

Thus, this is the first project to show in a controlled experiment significant differences in average growth rate of all children in communities receiving specific nutrition and health inputs: Regression analysis on a sub-sample of 180 children on whom exact dietary measurements were obtained showed a strong correlation between dietary intake and improved anthropometric status. Psychomotor development was found to have been directly affected by past nutritional status.

Results Pertaining to Morbidity

(i) There was significant reduction in the average duration of episodes of infectious diseases in health care villages as compared to villages without health care; and

(ii) In health care villages each episode of diarrhoeal disease was reduced on the average by two days, lower respiratory tract infections by 1-1/2 days and skin infection by 1-1/2 days in comparison with villages without health care.

Results Pertaining to Mortality: The mortality figures come from the final report of the Narangwal Population Project, since reports from the nutrition project do not show mortality rates for different time periods.

(i) Infant mortality rates declined considerably in the nutrition and medical care villages between 1970-71 and 1972-73 (Pre intervention IMR or 129 per 1000 came down to 107 per thousand during 1972-73);

(ii) In the nutrition care villages, the improvements occurred entirely in the neo-natal period while in the medical care villages rates in both the neo natal and post natal periods declined; and

(iii) The combined nutrition and medical care villages surprisingly did not experience a mortality decline although in 1970-71 they had the lowest overall levels of infant mortality recorded. The 1-3 year olds mortality rate in these villages was higher than in other treatment groups (i.e. nutrition and medical care clusters separately) although substantially lower than in the control group. Perhaps, the addition of family planning activities to the responsibilities of family health workers in the combined service villages resulted in a lower level of child nutrition and medical care in these villages than in the other two treatment groups.

2.2.2 The Tamilnadu International Nutrition Project (TINP), started with the assistance of World Bank in 1980 aimed at evolving a replicable model of a nutrition programme which would, through adopting a risk approach, be cost effective, efficient and promote better nutrition and health practices within the families. At present the project covers a total of 9 districts in the state, covering population of 17.3 million. Services are provided through 8965 Community Nutrition Centres (CNCs) and 2723 health sub-centres. Two innovative features are the hallmark of TINP. First, child beneficiaries are identified and monitored through a monthly growth monitoring system based in villages. Secondly, supplementation is continued only as long as required *i.e.*, till the child makes adequate nutritional recovery. In the third phase, nutrition education is imparted to the mothers for longer lasting improvement in health care practices of the family. The CNC is usually housed in a rented accommodation, manned by a Community Nutrition Worker and a helper. The CNW is a local resident mother of a healthy child. The CNW weighs children every month on a Tansi scale. Weight is recorded in a register as well as a card at the centre. Another growth card is kept by the mother on which the readings are entered at the time of weighing or later during house visits by CNW. The special feature of the growth card is that the divisions for recording weight are for 100 gms in consonance with the sensitivity of the weighing scale. An important issue related to the use of growth cards is the extent to which they are used as an educational tool. An evaluation agency found that most mothers interviewed can interpret the trends of growth lines. Some of them actually used the growth card to explain the effect of diarrhoea on growth.

The action response to deviant growth in a child ranges from active surveillance, supplementary feeding, referral and finally education to the mother. Children who have growth faltering but not to the extent that they need to be put on supplementary nutrition are given added attention by the CNW.

Supplementary feeding is indicated for children with PEM grade III and IV and those with no weight gain or weight loss. The minimum duration of supplementary feeding is discontinued when the child moves into grade II or I or following a weight gain of at least 500 gms registered over one month in 6-12 months age group and 3 months in the 13-26 months age group.

Strengths of Growth-monitoring Content can be summarised as strong motivation among leaders. GM was added to a pre-existing primary health care programme; high community awareness; active participation by mothers; CNW belonging to the target community itself. And lastly, the most unique strategy of TINP is formation of Childrens' Working Groups (CWG). The idea behind CWGs was initiated by field workers, and is an illustration of the flexibility of the system and stress on initiative and creativity at the grass root level. The CWGs are deployed for motivating and educating mothers on health and nutrition. They work through folk theatre, drama, school and festivals.

2.2.3 *Indo-Dutch Project for Child Welfare*

Found its origin in the personal interest that was shown by the Queen of Netherlands. The Netherlands Foundation was formally established in 1966, but the Indo-Dutch project was launched in 1970.

The Basic objective of the project is to improve the quality of life by enlisting community support for the overall development of children of the age of 0-16 years through an integrated programme of health, nutrition and education. Though initially work began in rural area of Chevalla Block in Andhra Pradesh, the urban project in the municipal area of Hyderabad city covering two blocks in ward 20 was added in 1976. Delivery of GM services was arranged by deploying mobile health units and starting 'creches' for under 36 months children of working mothers. While the mobile health unit provided antenatal, postnatal, immunization and health care of malnourished children the 'creches' included nutrition education to the mothers on an individualized basis.

A longitudinal study conducted by the project nutritionist revealed that vis-a-vis a well matched control group the mean increase in weight in the 'creche' children was more than the control group children. Similarly increase in height and mid-arm circumference were significantly greater in 'creche' children vis-a-vis the control group. This could be under the impact of supplementary nutrition to children and nutrition education to their mothers. The education service to the mothers also raised their awareness about nutritions food, importance of hygiene and better child rearing practices. However, on the negative side, the results of mental development show that the impact of 'creche' was not very encouraging when compared with the control group. That could be attributed to the need of better trained and more qualified helpers as also educative toys.

2.2.4 *The Kasa Project*

Aided by the WHO and started in 1971 was one of the early projects that devised the system of village level social workers on a part time basis to organise delivery of health care and nutrition services to the underfives at their door-step even in the remotest locations.

The Kasa Project, situated north of Bombay, started with the objective of studying the feasibility of a system for delivering integrated health, nutrition and family planning services to young children and their mothers, in which existing health-nutrition programmes and personnel of the government were utilized, community support is developed, persons from the community were used to serve as link workers in providing services to all. The project established a new system for delivering health and nutrition services through a domiciliary cum clinic outreach. The salient features included: integration of nutrition and health services by promotion of adequate growth of underfives through health education, immunization, treatment of illness including oral rehydration of diarrhoeal cases, provision of special care for 'at-risk' children and the most needy; the development of simplified technology and methodology which have now been found suitable for wider use, such as weighing scales having calibration in vernacular and protective cheap tin caps; swing seats for weighing children, shoulder bags; very simple weight charts; plastic overlay stencils for assessing nutritional grades, comprehensive but simple mothers' charts; index cards for assignment' identification and evaluation and community participation through the contributions in kind by the people—Shah and Junnarkar (1973).

The scope and coverage of the project which was operated in the governmental set up was quite wide. Yet community health workers were employed on a part-time basis. Using full-time workers involves high expenditure, transfers, associations, unions and many such problems. Second important lesson from this project is that the workers should concentrate on children and women as in these vulnerable segments of community, the morbidity and mortality is very high. Their efforts should not get diluted with excessive work of malaria control and running clinics. The emphasis should be on domiciliary approach for promotional and preventive activities.

2.2.5 *Comprehensive Rural Health Project Jamkhed*

It is an outstanding illustration of local organisations engaged in voluntary efforts. As suggested by the title of the project, its activities extend well beyond health care of underfives but for the present purposes, quite naturally only the relevant ones have been presented here. The project was initiated in Jamkhed, a small town 50 miles from the city of Ahmednagar in Maharashtra—by two rural service oriented doctors, namely, Dr. and Dr. (Mrs) R.S. Arole in October 1970. Operating under the umbrella of Marathi Mission which also provided the initial financial support, a dispensary was started in what was once a shed of a veterinary hospital. The target population is scattered over more than 30 villages. An individual village is considered a unit for health services. Each village has a health worker VHW, who is a well liked resident of the community, usually a woman. Jamkhed has a well equipped health centre. Most villages are within a distance of 16 km. from Jamkhed. A mobile health team supervises the VHWs on a weekly basis. Thus about 40,000 people get intensive care while an additional 40,000 people avail themselves of the diagnostic and curative services available at the centre. All the needy underfives are given one nutritious meal a day and complete immunization. Antenatal and postnatal care of every mother is provided by the VHW. Four visits are undertaken by the nurse during the course of one pregnancy to give tetanus toxoid injections and to decide on hospital or domicilliary delivery services is the responsibility of the VHW who is trained to conduct deliveries and recognise complications. Family planning services follow a cafeteria approach with emphasis on spacing. In each village a local woman is selected to work as a VHW and she is responsible for the health activities in her village. Her role is to undertake preventive and promotional health work and to give simple primary health care. The VHW is given intensive training in health education, the care of underfives and maternity cases. Being part of the community, she is familiar with existing social, economic and cultural problems and is able to communicate with community members in a manner understood by them. Another advantage of her being a local person is that she is available to the community any time during the day or night. The basic principles of training imparted to VHWs are minimal direct teaching, maximization of experiential learning, utilization of training materials developed from locally available and relevant materials and phased, on the job training. After selection, the VHWs undergo a one week orientation training at Jamkhed. There are four lectures in a day—two in the morning and two in the evening. Each session lasts for half an hour only. That is the maximum direct teaching resorted to. The classroom climate is always informal. Considerable use is made of audio-visual aids. Due emphasis is laid on raising the self-esteem, self-confidence and hope of success amongst trainees through positive reinforcements. This indeed is an on-going process and does not end with the orientation period. After the initial orientation, the VHWs are posted in their villages and asked to undertake such tasks as organising feeding programmes, convincing the people of utility of immunization, ante-natal service etc. Thereafter they report to headquarters once a week for discussion of causes, collection of medicines, deposit proceeds of sales of medicines and receiving instructions for next week. During the second spell of their training they observe and investigate birth and death cases. The lessons are built around the reported incidents. During the next six months emphasis remains on preventive work. Only after six months they are expected to handle primary curatology.

This Magsaysay Award project has its strengths in scientific training of personnel, an inbuilt concurrent evaluation and monitoring system; a strong community involvement evident from community volunteers identifying their health problems, providing space for clinic, helping in immunization and family planning campaigns, help in running community kitchens for underfives etc.

2.2.6 *Child In Need Institute (CINI) Project, West Bengal*

The project delivers a comprehensive package of primary health services in which growth monitoring is a pivotal activity. The nodal point of GM are a series of 10 clinics serving both rural and urban areas covering a population of 74,000. There is no home based GM service. The Service Package includes GM service at clinic level; home based rehydration therapy for diarrhoea cases; immunization of underfives and pregnant mothers; vitamin A deficiency prophylaxis programme; simple health care of underfives, pregnant and lactating mothers, health and nutrition education and rehabilitation of severely malnourished children. In case, a child suffers weight loss an assessment of the underlying causes is made and the mother is advised accordingly. The mother is also encouraged to buy supplementary food packets provided at subsidized rates. However, there is no follow up at the domicilliary level but the child and the mother are advised to visit the clinic every fortnight.

In case of grade II malnutrition cases, again, an attempt is made to identify causes and a referral service is provided. The follow up of severely malnourished children is quite good. On the negative side, it may be mentioned that at CINI no special note is taken of inadequate or no weight gain cases as evaluated by a UNICEF (1986) sponsored team.

Strengths of the project can be summarized as active involvement of mothers in discharging GM service; in-service continuous education to health workers; good rapport between mothers and health workers;

frequent use of audio-visual aids in training; periodic revision of nutrition and health education messages; active involvement of mothers in developing the educational messages through communication workshops.

2.2.7 *The Kangzha Project*

Which was implemented in mid-70s in 30 schools (total students 30,0000) of Central Kerela, made successful attempts to strengthen the role of school teachers as health workers. Recognizing the role of school children and teachers as change agents in social development, a three-tier approach was adopted in which each school with a trained teacher had a health unit providing simple curative services-peripheral tier. These school units in turn were linked to primary health centre-tier 2; and a referral hospital tier 3. The teachers and pupils, with the support of PHC staff, participated in the village health programme with the following aim for each school unit:

— immunization of 10 children under five years.
— organisation of compost and soakage farm manure pits for 5 houses.
— Imparting simple nutrition messages to 10 families.

The Kangzha Project demonstrated that the participation by pupils in the under-fives' health promotion programme sensitized the school children to the health needs of their own younger brothers and sisters and they became effective promoters of health in a development perspective. The pilot project proved that school teachers and students are a high potential resource for PHC through peoples' participation.

2.2.8 *Malwani Project*

Another interesting small scale health programme was the Malwani Project started in 1976 when the Seth GS Medical School, Bombay worked in collaboration with the municipal school staff in low income suburbs of Malwani on the outskirts of Bombay. For the children in Malwani slums, it was an interesting way of using their long summer vacation and for the health professionals it meant a field practice area for developing methods for delivery of primary health care. The maximum number of child voluntary health workers (617) were trained in 1978-79. The children were initiated through role play, discussions, demonstrations and pictorial teaching tools. The trained children assisted the health staff in identifying the needs of the community and bringing them to the attention of PHCs.

The role of teachers lay in identifying suitable children for the said role and assisting them.

Results obtained were quite encouraging indeed. The immunization coverage increased from 20 to 90 per cent. Hundreds of cases, including those of vitamin 'A' deficiency, T.B., Scabies, Malnutrition etc. were brought to the health centre. The success is attributed to the high commitment of project personnel; and the rapport between medical college and school teachers.

2.2.9 *Action Research for Community Health (ARCH), Mangrol Project*

A group of individuals of diverse background and training got together in Mangrol, Gujarat for diverse developmental work in the areas of health, education, rehabilitation of Narmada oustees and disaster relief etc. The main strategy of growth-monitoring was to impart skills and knowledge to health assistants drawn from the same community so that they can run and maintain the essential components of health services on their own, such as:

- growth-monitoring of underfives,
- handling of nutritional emergencies, and
- training the second generation of community health workers.

Identification of high risk children and their treatment; teaching mothers correct breast-feeding and weaning practices; oral rehydration therapy for diarrhoeal cases; comprehensive immunization; pre-natal care by identifying high risk mothers; propagation of correct infant feeding and infant care practices etc. were the major activities of growth-monitoring.

2.2.10 *Ghatla Project by Tata Institute of Social Sciences*

The project was initially started by the department of Social and Preventive Medicine, L.T.M.G. Hospital in 1973 and soon later field work students of medical and psychiatric social work from TISS joined them.

The broad goal was to reach out to Ghatla community and help the people utilize the hospital facilities so that they move towards total health *i.e.*, physical, social, emotional and mental.

Health Care of underfives was accorded the top priority it deserves. An underfives' clinic was set up which provided the services of routine medical check up and necessary treatment; Immunization against Small

Pox, Polio, Cholera and Typhoid; referrals; and high protein supplementary nutrition. Secondly, the mothers of underfives, through group work practice, were imparted knowledge of balanced diet, sickness care, importance of immunization and emotional needs of underfives, and how to use the nutritional supplements. The women were encouraged to talk in the group on subjects close to their heart *e.g.* how did they handle food fads in children, and what were their cultural beliefs affecting health of underfives etc. Secondly, besides education, recreation was an important part of group activities *e.g.* haldi-kumkum, picnic, bhajan sessions etc.

Important Lessons: Lobo Marie (1977) has analysed following lessons from Ghatla Project:

1. Know the culture in which work is to be done.
2. Learn to recognise those new beliefs which can be readily incorporated into the existing culture.
3. Take advantage of the pragmatic nature of people *i.e.* have short term achievable goals.
4. Use existing leadership whenever feasible.
5. Select the more progressive members for further teaching and training.
6. Ask payment for services whenever such payment is applicable.
7. One should equip oneself with knowledge and skill which will be necessary as one has to take the leadership role in the community, initially.
8. One should not expect automatic acceptance from the community: it has to be earned over a period of time with consistent and persistent efforts.
9. As Prof. N.F. Kaikabad says, 'one should always hope for the best even when every thing seems to be going wrong and the horizon appears bleak. Remember, the darkest hours are always, before the dawn of the new day, and this holds true for the work in the community too.

2.2.11 *Integrated Child Development Services (ICDS) Scheme*

It is one of the few programmes of child health any-where in the developing world which has made any significant and permanent improvement in the life of a nation. The scheme was initiated by the government of India on a pilot basis in 1975, in collaboration with UNICEF.

The Specific Goals: Reduce the incidence of low birth weight and severe malnutrition among children:

— bring down the mortality and morbidity rates among children 0-6 years old;
— reduce school dropout rates through early stimulation programme for children 3-6 years old;
— lay the foundation for psychological and social development of under six children; and
— enhance the capability of the mother to look after the health and nutrition needs of the child.

The heart of the ICDS is the 'anganwadi' — literally the courtyard, which is used as a centre for information and help with child care. The front-line worker is the Anganwadi Worker (AWW), who is usually selected by the community and serves a population of about 1000. About 20 AWWs are supervised by an Anganwadi Supervisor (AWS). The Child Development Officer (CDPO) is officer-in-charge of 100 Anganwadis *i.e.* one block. The AWW is assisted by a helper, who is often a local traditional birth attendant, but could be anyone else also. The rest of the health team consists of Auxilliary Nurse Midwife (ANMs), Lady Health Visitors (LHVs) and the Medical Officers of the block Primary Health Centre.

Monthly weighing is one of the job responsibilities of an AWW. Children under 3 years who do not visit the anganwadi are weighed at home. The AWW usually combines this task with imparting of one-to-one nutrition education to the mother. Secondly, the growth cards of all beneficiary children in the form of a book are maintained at the anganwadi. In many parts of the country, initially the AWWs used a register to record weights first and then plot the graphs. But now-a-days with increasing skill and confidence, plotting is done directly on the cards. Mothers do not keep the growth chart; it is designed more for the AWW's use.

In addition to growth-monitoring services, the under six beneficiaries of ICDS scheme also receive periodic medical examination and treatment, referral, comprehensive immunization, supplementary nutrition which includes pregnant and lactating mothers as well. Nutrition education on an informal basis is also provided to the mothers of under six.

Whether we speak of strengths or the drawbacks of the programme, it would have to be very much in a generalized form. It is not possible to cover the individual or even the regional variations in this regard here.

The extensive coverage by the ICDS itself is an important strength in the context of a developing nation. The services of periodic weighing, immunization and supplementary nutrition are delivered as per schedule.

The partial objectives of periodic weighing namely—to determine the nutritional status, eligibility for supplementary feeding and need for medical attention are also served well. The follow up action once grade III or IV malnutrition sets in is quite effective. The effected children are put on weekly observations and weighed at home by the AWWS, intensive nutrition education is given to the mother, a separate follow up card and double the amount of supplementary feeds are provided. The special cards for cases of severe malnutrition are filled accurately in most cases (which facilitates follow up action).

The most serious drawback of ICDS scheme lies in its training of AWWs with regard to use of growth cards for promotional aspects of growth monitoring. The AWWs usually still lack in recognising early growth faltering and consequently their response action gets delayed causing further deterioration of the child's nutritional status. Similarly, their understanding and interpretation of growth curves is weak. Few possess the knowledge and skill necessary to enlist optimum community participation. Lastly, there could be improvements in the space in which Anganwadi functions and the quality of supplementary nutrition or the educational material used.

2.2.12 *Ashish Gram Rachana Trust, Pachod, Maharashtra*

The project was launched in 1977 in Aurangabad district of Maharashtra and it covered a population of about 60,000. Besides, GM and nutritional surveillance of underfives the services included MCH, health and nutrition education as well as an environmental and social forestry programme. The target area is divided into 12 sub-centres, each with an approximate population of 5000. The sub-centre represents an administrative area and not a physically fixed centre facility. A sub centre area is served by one male and one female multi-purpose worker (MPW). The worker conducts house to house visits instead of delivering outpatient services from a fixed centre. Services provided by the MPWs include: GM of underfives; nutritional surveillance and education; census enumeration; detection of pregnant women and record keeping. The MPW does not dispense curative drugs but may diagnose illness and request the peripheral health worker to prescribe drugs from her kit. There are two cadres of community based health workers: the CHW and the *dai* (Traditional Birth attendant). provision of maternal and neo-natal care is the exclusive duty of the *dai* which encompasses monitoring of tetanus toxoid vaccination, iron and folic acid supplements, intra-natal and post-natal care. The CHW carries the responsibility of imparting health education, motivating mothers to utilize health services and treating common ailments.

This project has evolved an innovative strategy for health delivery services through creation of "Health Posts". Four ANMs are transported everyday in a vehicle to 4 neighbouring villages. Health care services are rendered from any fixed village facility, such as a panchayat building, an Anganwadi or the residence of CHW or MPW. Each village is covered 2 times a week and immunization is administered once a month. In this way, the costs required for maintaining a daily fixed centre are reduced and at the same time, due to the mobility factor CHDP can cover a large population. Further, the strategy involves the creation and use of a network of community helpers in the so-called "peer-to-peer" out-reach model. Professionals train community women in aspects of pre-natal and child care, these women then teach parents how to care for their children and also how to make appropriate use of available health and education facilities.

2.2.13 *SEWA—Rural, Jhagadia, Gujarat*

SEWA—Rural, an acronym for Society for Education, Welfare and Action was initiated by a group of young doctors and other professionals at Jhagadia in Bharuch district of Gujarat state. It started in October 1980 with hospital services and later expanded into other developmental activities. It now provides a comprehensive and integrated package of health and development services to the predominantly tribal population of Jhagadia block. The society's programme can be classified into those that are directly medical and health related and those activities with the broader aim of improving general socio-economic conditions. In the former category, basic curative, preventive and promotive health care is made available at a 70 bed hospital. Environmental improvement activities, afforestation, youth training, and women's income generation activities comprise the second category.

SEWA—Rural functions on the principles of social service, scientific approach and spiritual faith and has conviction in the effectiveness of close collaboration between the voluntary agency, the local community and the government. The organisation and its functioning run on scientific lines characterised by use of modern managerial concepts like well defined job descriptions, performance appraisal, feed back, research and an on-going internal evaluation. Policy making staff and field level workers meet regularly for exchange of ideas and experience which contributes significantly towards smooth implementation of planned programme. Also, the project supervisors who provide the link between the board members and the field staff play a key role to ensure formulation of realistic policies and programmes.

In 1984, the state government of Gujarat handed over 10 primary health sub-centres to SEWA—Rural to meet the health needs of 40 villages in Jhagadia block. The society has also assumed responsibility for running 45 'Anganwadis' under the state sponsored Integrated Child Development Scheme. The following statistics speak volumes for the child health care activities of the Community Health Project:

Parameter	1981 (Base-line)	1991
IMR	172/1000	100.8/1000
MMR	13%	7.4%
Ante-natal Care Coverage	50%	85%
Trained personnel at delivery	25%	90%
BCG vaccine coverage	33%	96%
Measles vaccine	0	87%
Polio	9%	90%
DPT	7%	88%

(The above data was compiled during a field visit)

2.2.14 *Mini Health Centres of Voluntary Health Services Tiruporur Block Chingleput Dist. Tamilnadu*

The Project started in 1977 now covers a total population of more than 160,000. One Mini Health Centre (MHC) caters to the health needs of about 5000 people. The regular activities of the centre make a comprehensive package of ante-natal care, post-natal care, growth monitoring of under-fives, immunization, nutritional assessment, treatment and surveillance.

The key ingredient of the VHS approach to health care was the involvement of the community in the planning, execution and even financing of the MHC. Community participation in the planning process is a difficult concept to enforce. Keeping this in mind VHS set up local action committees which were responsible for generating awareness in the community that the MHC was very much a peoples' project in the successful running of which they had an integral stake.

At the execution stage, the community participated through having a say in actual location of MHC and in providing the building and furniture. Financial participation took the form of enrolment by the people as subscribers to a prepayment scheme conceived somewhat along the lines of health insurance or actual payment for services received by non-subscribers of modest amounts scheduled according to their capacity to pay.

The concept of pre-payment was hard to sell. In India, public health has been a government run and government subsidised operation. The community had to be educated to contribute a token amount towards the cost of maintenance of health records, basic immunization and routine health check up which would help to detect disease and identify remedial action. Next, the success of the MHC had to be demonstrated to the community before it could be actually convinced of subscriber enrolment.

2.2.15 *Extracts from A Research Study on "Food Dietary Intake and Feeding practices in Urban Slums in Visakhapatnam", Busi B.R. et al. (1987)*

Its a study of five slums in Visakhapatnam from which 113 families were randomly selected for assessment of dietary intakes. The family dietary intakes were obtained by interview method. The breast feeding practices and supplementary foods given to the underfives were also recorded. The per capita food consumption was estimated from the family's diet by the use of consumption co-efficients.

Results of Breast Feeding Patterns: It was observed that all children were breast fed till the end of first year. A gradual decrease was noted from then onwards with 25 per cent of females being breastfed till fourth year and 11 per cent of males continued upto fifth year.

Results of Supplementary Feeding Pattern: The supplementary feeding was mostly reported as biscuits and chocolates. Only 5 per cent were given baby foods like Farex before 1 year and 25 per cent were given cooked foods like idli and pogadalu. Additional milk was given to 40 per cent children below one year. The number, consuming milk dwindled rapidly with increase in age. There was no proper weaning at all. Mothers had a belief that as long as the child was on the breast, there was no need for supplementary foods.

Results of Diet Patterns in Families: It was observed that consumption of rice, dal, vegetables and fish was high in small families, and generally speaking consumption of these foods decreased with increasing family size. Consumption of milk was more or less small in all families size *i.e.*, about 18 to 22 ml; per day mostly in the form of tea. The diet of all families was deficient in calories, minerals and vitamins while only a few were deficient in proteins. The main cause of calorie deficiency was reported to be socio-economic.

2.2.16 *Extracts from a Research Study on "Nutritional Status of Preschool Children in Rural Hissar" by Kakker, S. et al. (1987)*

Hundred Children between one to five years of age were selected at random from 2 villages of Hissar district. The data regarding general information were collected by using a pretested and structured interview schedule from the parents of the selected children. Anthropometric measurements were recorded using standard techniques of Jellife (1966). The haemoglobin estimation was done by Winterobe (1958) method. The nutritional assessment of children was made by comparing their height and weight statistics for a particular age and sex with ICMR (1984) values.

Results of Anthropometric Measurements: Weight for age measure was used to determine the degree of malnutrition. Out of the 100 children under study only 18 per cent were normal; 38 per cent were in grade I; 31 per cent in grade II; 9 per cent in grade III and 4 per cent in grade IV of malnutrition. The mean height of the children in the study, surprisingly, was found to be higher than ICMR recommended values for a particular age and sex.

Results of Haemoglobin Estimation: Only 21.5 per cent children had haemoglobin levels between 9.0-11.0 gm/dl range. The majority *i.e.*, 56.96 per cent belonged to 7.0 to 8.9 gm/dl category; 18.99 per cent belonged to 5.0 to 6.9 gm/dl category; and 2.53 per cent belonged to below 5 gm/dl group. On the whole, the picture was quite gloomy considering the WHO standard of 11.0 gm/dl as the desirable level of haemoglobin for underfive children from poverty groups.

2.2.17 *Extract from a Research Study on "Perceived Morbidity, Medically Defined Morbidity, Population Typology and Its Relevance in Planning for Health Services" by Pathak M. et. al. (1985)*

The data used in the study pertains to previous general health surveys carried out in slums of Nagpur city and 43 villages around Saoner town. Morbidity data was analysed according to perception of illness and medically defined illness, to determine whether any association exists between perceived morbidity and medically defined morbidity. The study is based on the assumption that morbidity has a strong subjective element: many people feel ill when there is no clinical evidence to label them ill on one hand and many others who feel fit can have medically defined morbidity.

Results: x^2 test was used to determine any association between perceived morbidity and medically defined morbidity and was found to be highly significant at P<.001 level.

Comparison between perceived sickness rate and medically defined sickness rate for total population revealed only a small difference between the two *i.e.*, when perceived morbidity rate was 176.3 per thousand medically defined morbidity was only 138.1 per thousand.

However age-wise distribution of these rates showed that the medically defined illnesses are 2.24 and 3.6 times higher in infants and children of 1-5 year age group.

Therefore, if perceived sickness rate is used as an indicator for need level of health services, it would grossly underestimate the true need.

2.2.18 *Extract from a Research Study on "Survey of Anaemia in Children in Bombay" by Currimbhoy Z. and Phadke P. (1963)*

The report is based upon a study carried out in a hospital at Bombay. New born children and their mothers as well as children in the age group of 8 to 12 years were studied.

Major Findings

1. About 93 per cent of the infants were anaemic. The main causes for this were assigned as pre-maturity and breast feeding upto one year. It was observed however that upto 3 months haemoglobin was unaffected.
2. The haemoglobin level fell upto one year of age. The study recommended that to improve the haemoglobin level of children it is imperative that some iron nutrient be given to them right from the age of two to three months.

2.2.19 *Extracts from a Research Study on "Morbidity and Mortality in Preschool Children", Seminar Paper by Balgopal, R. et al. (1970)*

At a seminar in Madras organised by ICSW the authors presented a paper based on a survey by the noted nutritionist, Dr. Gopalan C. in 9 villages during 1951 under the aegis of peripheral paediatrics clinic of Institute of Child Health and Hospital for Children, Madras.

Major findings

1. 74 per cent children were not healthy.
2. Main causes of morbidity and mortality in preschool children

were assigned as: (1) malnutrition, and (2) acute chronic infections, many of which were caused by lowered resistance due to malnutrition and poor environmental hygiene.

Suggestions

The authors suggested both long-term and short-term plans to reduce morbidity and mortality. Health education for different categories of workers in health field, better sanitary conditions and protected water supply were suggested as the long-term measures. Supply of nutritive food and nutrition education to mothers were put forth as short-term measures. The authors also suggested setting up well planned and well staffed mother-craft centres in each state—thus advocating improvement of knowledge and practice of health care amongst mothers.

2.2.20 *Extract from a Research Study on "Morbidity and Mortality in Children" by Gandhi, V.K. (1963)*

The study pertains to 2476 cases admitted to children's ward of a hospital over a period of two years. The diagnosis was arrived at mainly by clinical means, laboratory investigations and radiological aids.

Major Findings

1. Morbidity and mortality incidences were highest during the first two years. 28.1 per cent cases under one year and 46.6 per cent cases between one and two years of age.
2. More male *i.e.*, 62.1 per cent children were brought for treatment as against only 37.9 per cent female children. This could possibly by a pointer towards greater attention received by male children from their parents vis-a-vis their female counter parts.
3. 69.5 per cent morbidity and 81.9 per cent mortality could be accounted for by respiratory, communicable, gastrointestinal and nervous system diseases.
4. About 60.9 per cent of total mortality occured within 24 hours of admission to hospital. Could this be due to the fact that children are usually brought for medical treatment only in the advanced stage of their illness?

3

THE BASELINE SURVEY

As reported earlier, the experimental study was carried out in three major stages, namely, the base-line survey; organising a package of health care and growth-monitoring activities for the study children; and imparting health education to the mothers of these children. This chapter presents the survey findings of 115 families residing in Harijanwas and Sardargram pockets of Pensionpura slums located in administrative ward number nineteen of Vadodara city. At the outset, it would be in order to briefly delineate the rationale behind the survey, other than indeed, the objective of identifying the target families. The researcher on account of her substantial field experience in slum community work and course teaching of 'Rural, Urban, Tribal Community Development' did have an insight that the intended study would not only be relevant but also a viable one. But for any scientific inquiry such 'insight' alone is inadequate. More so for an experimental study where-in empirical data must form the basis for the underlying assumptions leading to the study design. It has been observed that many projects fail to reach their goals because the following question has been inadequately considered: on, what basis and towards what end, will who do what to whom, for how long, with what effect and with what benefits?

The present survey addressed itself to the task of determining the demographic and socio-economic condition of the respondent families and also sought relevant information pertaining to certain factors closely related to the health of underfives *i.e.,* daily diet patterns, actual per day consumption of essential food items, incidence of pregnancy wastage and child mortality, utilization of ante-natal, natal, post-natal and family planning services, age at weaning and types of weaning foods given etc,.

The gleanings from the survey analysed for suitable statistical measures follow.

3.1 Religion, Caste, Mother Tongue and Native Place

Religion, Caste, Mother tongue and place of origin are some of the important cultural variables as far as health and illness in a society are concerned. Medical scientists have well established the close link between cultural factors and personal hygiene, nutrition, family planning, immunisation, child rearing, disposal of refuse and excreta, environmental sanitation, outlook on health and disease, propensity to seek timely

TABLE: 3.1 : Religion, Caste, Mother Tongue and Native Place

	Variable	Distribution	
		F	%
	Religion		
(i)	Hindu	106	92.17
(ii)	Christian	6	5.22
(iii)	Muslim	3	2.61
(iv)	Others	0	0.00
	Total	115	100.00
	Caste		
(i)	Harijan	51	44.35
(ii)	SC/ST other than Harijan	48	41.03
(iii)	Upper Castes	7	6.80
(iv)	Non-castes	9	7.82
	Total	115	100.00
	Mother Tongue		
(i)	Gujarati	85	73.91
(ii)	Marathi	15	13.05
(iii)	Hindi	6	5.22
(iv)	Any other	9	7.82
	Total	115	100.00
	Native Place		
(i)	Baroda district	65	56.41
(ii)	Gujarat State but not Baroda district.	18	15.82
(iii)	Outside Gujarat	32	27.77
	Total	115	100.00

medical care etc. or in short, the way of life. India being a traditional society, the study of these cultural factors becomes fundamental to our purpose.

In this study it was found that a vast majority of the families were Hindus 92.17 per cent followed by Christians 5.22 per cent, Muslims 2.61 per cent and 'Nil' reporting for 'any other' category. This meant that we had a near homogeneous population on the religion criterion which facilitated further health interventions. However, caste-wise distribution presented a heterogeneous picture, with Harijans or, the so called 'untouchables' making up for 44.35 per cent; schedule caste and schedule tribes other than Harijans adding upto 41.03 per cent; and the remaining being upper castes – 6.80 per cent and non-castes – 7.82 per cent. The upper caste families were mainly migrants from outside Gujarat, especially Rajputs and Thakurs from Rajasthan. Christians and Muslims were classified as non-castes since these religions do not have a caste system akin to Hindus.

Throughout the study we found that Harijans in comparison with other caste groups were invariably less participative in the intervention programmes. In fact, each time we had to be more persuasive in their case whereas others readily joined in. Harijans, having suffered severe social discrimination for centuries together, it was hardly surprising that they were sceptical about our work.

Based on the criterion of mother tongue our population was distributed as follows: Gujarati-73.91 per cent, Marathi-13.05 per cent, Hindi-5.22 per cent, 'Any other'-7.82 per cent. 'Any other' category included Punjabi, Sindhi, Tamil and Nepali. It was decided to prepare our audio-visual aids for the health education programme in Gujarati.

Regarding place of origin, study revealed that 56.41 per cent belonged to Baroda district, 15.82 per cent families hailed from within Gujarat but districts other than Baroda and close to one-thirds *i.e.*, 27.77 per cent had migrated from outside Gujarat. One can catch a glimpse of the cosmopolitan character of Vadodara city in the slum area too.

3.2 Family Type, Family Size and Food Consumption Units in a Family

In our study, under nuclear families we include those families where a couple and their un-married children were residing; while in joint families there were one or more additional members, related to the couple and living in the same household. Accordingly, there were 63.06 per cent nuclear families and the rest 36.92 per cent were joint; both figures being

TABLE: 3.2 : Family Type, Family Size and Food Consumption Units (in a family)

	Variable		Distribution F	%
	Family Type			
(i)	Nuclear		73	63.07
(ii)	Joint		42	36.93
		Total	155	100.00
	Family Size			
(i)	2—3		18	15.65
(ii)	4—5		64	55.66
(iii)	6—7		27	23.47
(iv)	8—9		6	5.22
(v)	10—11		0	0.00
		Total	115	100.00
	Food Consumption Units			
(i)	2.0—3.0		30	26.08
(ii)	3.1—4.0		33	28.69
(iii)	4.1—5.0		32	27.82
(iv)	5.1—6.0		14	12.19
(v)	6.1—7.0		6	5.22
(vi)	7.1—8.0		0	0.00
		Total	115	100.00

Mean Family Size: 4.91 members; S.D. = 1.43 members

Mean Consumption Units in a family; 4.03; S.D. = 1.18.

typical of urban living.

Family type is an important structural variable which has a bearing on the present study at least in two distinct ways. First, the upbringing, health care and socialization that a child receives is characteristically different amongst nuclear and joint families. Second, in joint families decision-making power gravitates more towards elders in the family vis-a-vis the nuclear families where this power is shared by the couple equitably or otherwise. The study of these trends was essential towards working out our strategies of conducting the health education programme for mothers.

Family size, once again, affects the socialization process for a child in the family. We have also used this data extensively to compute per capita monthly incomes, food consumption units in a family and actual per day consumption of essential food items. In our study, mean family size was found to be 4.91 with a standard deviation of 1.43 members. This is slightly lower than that of mean family size of 5.0 members found in recent study of services areas of Baroda Citizens Council according to Rajyaguru (1988). Earlier, Parikh (1982) in his city level study of Baroda slum dwellers has mentioned a mean family size of 4.95 members, closer to this study.

Table 3.2 depicts that there were 15. 65 per cent families having 2 or 3 members; 55.65 per cent having 4 or 5 members; 23.47 per cent having 6 to 7 members and another 5.21 per cent having 8 or 9 members.

In recent years, the concept of food consumption units in a family has been developed to facilitate studies on nutritional status, consumption patterns and measuring standard of living. There are varying ways in which the consumption units are computed by different scholars and researchers. For our purpose, the formula developed by Djurfeldt and Lindberg (1975) for a study of introduction of western medicine in a Tamilnadu village has been used. According to the authors, if the age composition of the members of a household are taken into account when measuring consumption patterns, the food consumption units are calculated by counting an adult as one unit and other members in relation to this as follows:

Age of individual	*Counted as*
1—3 years	1/4 consumption unit
4—7 years	1/2 consumption unit
8—14 years	3/4 consumption unit
15—59 years	1 consumption unit
60 and above	3/4 consumption unit

Applying the above formula, the mean food consumption units per household was found to be 4.03 with a standard deviation of 1.18. Parikh (1982) in his earlier referred city level study of Baroda slum dwellers found this mean to be 3.81 per household. Indeed it needs to be mentioned here that Parikh has based his computations on a different formula. Table 3.2 depicts that there were 26.08 per cent having 3.1 to 4.0; 27.82 per cent having 4.1 to 5.0; 12.19 per cent having 5.1 to 6.0; and the remaining 5.22 per cent having 6.1 to 7.0.

3.3 Education, Occupation and Income

Observations that health and disease are not equally distributed in social classes have been reported for over a century. Individuals in the upper classes have a longer life expectancy, less mortality and better health and nutritional status than those in the lower classes. Secondly, there are startling differences in the utilisation of medical and health services in different social classes. Individuals in the lower social classes have been found to make less use of hospital facilities, consult the doctors less often and are less likely to utilise preventive health services like immunisation, ante natal and post natal care. Or in short, individuals in lower social classes are less health conscious as compared with those in the upper classes.

Education, occupation and income have been considered to be the most important variables of socio-economic stratification and the three aspects are highly intercorrelated too. Hollingshead in USA developed a scale using education, occupation and the residential address in lieu of income. In India, socio-economic status measuring scales by Kuppuswamy (1976) for urban areas and Pareek and Kulshrestha (1975) for rural and urban areas are better known.

The first mentioned determinant of socio-economic status, namely Education helps individuals in developing values, skills and abilities of various kinds. This in turn affects the performance of their roles as mothers, home-makers and fathers etc.

Table 3.3A depicts the educational status of adult males and females in the families studied. In keeping with all India trends educational level of men was much higher than women.

In the first category of illiterates there were 29.26 per cent males and 68.14 females. Correspondingly it is implied that literacy rate for men was 70.75 per cent; for Females-31.86 per cent; and the combined literacy

TABLE: 3.3A : Educational Status of the Adult Males and Females

Educational		Distribution of Males		Distribution of Females	
		F.	%	F.	%
(i)	Illiterate	43	29.26	92	68.14
(ii)	Primary i.e. up to 5th Std.	46	31.29	23	17.04
(iii)	Secondary i.e. up to 6th to 9th Std.	41	27.89	11	8.15
(iv)	Higher Secondary i.e. 10th to 12th Std.	17	11.56	8	5.93
v)	College or University education	0	0.00	1	0.74
	Total	147	100.00	135	100.00

level was 51.8 per cent. Rajyaguru (1988: 28) in a study of service areas of Baroda Citizens Council has reported literacy rates of men, women and combined as 74 per cent, 36 per cent and 55 per cent respectively. Parikh (1982) in a broader city level study of slum reported literacy levels as 73.28 per cent for males, 36.11 per cent as total literacy level of slum dwellers. It can be seen that in the present study literacy levels in each category are slightly lower as compared to both other studies.

In the second category, namely 'Primary' we included all those adults who had studied upto standard fifth. Accordingly, 31.29 per cent males and 17.04 per cent females were placed here.

The third category of 'Secondary' included 27.89 per cent men and 8.15 per cent women who had received education upto sixth, seventh, eighth or ninth standard.

There were 11.56 per cent men and 5.93 per cent women in the category of 'Higher Secondary' which included those individuals who were educated upto tenth, eleventh or twelfth standard.

Quite interestingly, in the last category 'college or university education' there was 'nil' reporting by men and 0.74 per cent (1 woman) of affirmative response by women. This lady had received two years of college education but not completed degree studies.

Occupational status can be a significant predictor of human behaviour because occupational groups vary widely, in terms of norms and values which either sanction or restrict the level and quality of participation

TABLE: 3.3B : Occupational Status of Head of Household

Category of Employment	Distribution	
	F.	%
(i) Unemployed	9	7.82
(ii) Self-employed	19	16.53
(iii) Non-Govt. employee	53	46.09
(iv) Govt. employee	34	29.56
	115	100.00

TABLE: 3.3C : Occupational Status of Lady of the Household (LOH)

Category of Employment	Distribution	
	F.	%
(i) House-wife	73	63.48
(ii) Self-employed	7	6.08
(iii) Employed earning	35	30.44
	115	100.00

in various activities by individuals in their homes or larger society. In lay terms, we often differentiate between 'blue collared workers' and 'white collared workers' more on the basis of their vastly different life styles.

For instance, a lower division clerk and a skilled or semi skilled industrial worker may have similar incomes (at times the latter may even be better paid) but their living standards are different in many ways because the former hardly ever reside in slums.

There are various ways in which occupations are classified. For our purpose in case of men we had four categories, *viz.*, 'unemployed', 'self-employed', 'non-government employee', and 'government employee'. Corresponding distribution for each of the categories above was 7.82 per cent, 16.53 per cent, 46.09 per cent and 29.56 per cent respectively. In the case of women there were only three categories *viz.*, 'housewife', 'self-employed', and 'employed earning'. The placement of women in each category was 63.48 per cent, 6.08 per cent and 30.44 per cent respectively. There are 36.52 per cent women engaged in gainful employment in addition to discharging of their regular housewifely roles. It is surmised that their role performance as mothers would be different than the remaining 63.50 per cent women who were pure housewives.

It is essentially the urban poor who are constrained to live in urban slums. In this study we have selected the parameter of monthly per capita income (PCI) for measuring income levels for two specific reasons. First, monthly PCI gives a clear picture of an individual's purchasing power or access to consumer, capital or luxury goods, (rather than family income). Secondly, a city level organisation, Baroda Citizens Council (BCC) has defined urban poverty in terms of PCI per month. For understanding the economic situation of study families we too have adopted the BCC concept according to which individuals having PCI of Rs. 100 or less per month

TABLE: 3.3D : Per Capita Monthly Incomes

Income range in Rs.	Distribution	
	F.	%
(i) 100 or less	32	27.82
(ii) 101 to 150	44	38.27
(iii) 151 to 200	22	19.13
(iv) 201 to 300	11	9.56
(v) 301 and above	6	5.22
	115	100.00

Mean per Capita Monthly Income = Rs. 148.35

S.D. = Rs. 77.6

are placed below poverty line. More specifically about the present study, the mean PCI per month was found to be Rs. 148.35 with a standard deviation of Rs. 77.6. High S.D. value is accepted because there was wide variation between the lowest reported PCI of Rs. 20 per month and the highest reported being Rs. 440 per month. According to a BCC report (1988: 31) mean PCI per month for its service area slum families was found to be Rs. 115. This suggests that the economic situation of the study families was considerably higher as compared to their compatriots else where in the city.

Table 3.3D depicts that there were 27.82 per cent families below 'poverty line' *i.e.*, with PCI of Rs. 100 or less per month; 38.27 per cent families in the second category of Rs. 101 to 150; 19.13 per cent placed in third category of Rs. 151 to 200; 9.56 per cent in the fourth category of Rs. 201 to 300 and only 5.22 per cent in the fifth category of Rs. 301 and above. Later tables numbered 3.4 and 3.5 on 'Ownership of household goods, other assets' and 'Indebtedness and saving habits' describe the economic situation further.

3.4 Ownership of Household Goods, other Assets

The study of this aspect not only lends further insight into the economic situation but it also served another important purpose. This alongwith study of 'housing, access to public utilities and environment' presented later helped us get a clearer understanding of their life styles which paved the way for constructing a 'situation practical' health education programme

TABLE: 3.4 Ownership of Household Goods and other Assets
A Multiple response Table

Item		Distribution F	Distribution %
(i)	House	107	93.00
(ii)	Cattle	13	11.30
(iii)	Land	25	21.73
(iv)	Cycle	82	71.30
(v)	Rickshaw and motorised Vehicle	8	6.95
(vi)	Furniture	82	77.30
(vii)	Radio/Transistor	61	53.04
(viii)	Tape Recorder	23	20.00
(ix)	T.V. Set	5	4.34
(x)	Any Other	19	16.52

for mothers of treatment group.

Table 3.4, understandably is a multi-response table depicting possession of physical assets. The lived in house was the commonest commodity owned *i.e.*, 93.0 per cent families had their own house. Further, they enjoy a fair sense of security of tenure because their locality, at least at present is in no imminent danger of eviction. Next, popular items were 'cycle' and 'furniture items' like a cot, chairs, a small table etc. Both categories were mentioned by 71.30 per cent families. 53.04 per cent families owned radios or transistors. This was the single most used means of mass media as none of the residents subscribed for newspaper as is typical of slum living 21.73 per cent owned land in their place of origin either as singular or joint owners, 20.0 per cent owned tape recorders and during our data collection many times we heard English pop music in passing. Cattle, *i.e.*, goats in all cases were owned by 11.30 per cent families who used goat milk. Rickshaw and motorised vehicles like mopeds were owned by 6.95 per cent; former as a means of living and the latter as a luxury item. At the time of inquiry 4.34 per cent owned TV sets but during our intervention we witnessed rapid additions of more sets. In 'any other' category, the investigators were instructed to include items like cupboards, clocks, fans etc. As such 16.52 per cent were placed in this category.

3.5 Indebtedness and Savings

The upper social classes harbour certain common notions about the poor. One, that the poor are invariably in debt. Two, that the unscruplous moneylender takes undue advantages of their hapless situation and "bleeds them white". Three, that the poor as a class lack futuristic vision. Neither do they believe in saving for a "rainy day" nor do they feel the necessity to save for acquiring some assets like a house, vehicle or higher education of children. Four, incapacity of the poor to save-since they spend more than 90 per cent of their income on purchasing food alone, is the other side of the notion "three" stated above. We queried into these aspects to ascertain how far the above ideas were tenable in case of families under study.

Table 3.5 shows while 60 per cent families were indebted yet a significant proportion *i.e.*, 40 per cent were free of debt. In the former category a large majority *i.e.*, 33.33 per cent had taken "Small loans", of rupees less than 1000 and another 15.94 per cent had dues between rupees 1001 to 2000. 26.09 per cent families had taken medium sized loans of amounts between rupees 2001 to 3000. On the higher side, 4.34 per cent

TABLE: 3.5 : Indebtedness and Savings

Variable			Distribution F	%
	Whether family is in debt?			
(i)	Yes		69	60.00
(ii)	No		46	40.00
		Total	115	100.00
	Amount of debt			
(i)	Less than Rs. 1000		23	33.33
(ii)	Rs. 1001—2000		11	15.95
(iii)	Rs. 2001— 3000		18	26.09
(iv)	Rs. 3001—4000		3	4.34
(v)	Rs. 4001—5000		9	13.05
(vi)	Above Rs. 5000		5	7.24
		Sub-total	69	100.00
	Sources of debt			
(i)	Friends and relations		25	36.24
(ii)	Co-operative societies		14	20.28
(iii)	Employer		15	21.74
(iv)	Money-lender		15	21.74
		Sub-total	69	100.00
	Whether family saves regularly?			
(i)	Yes		25	21.74
(ii)	No		90	78.26
		Total	115	100.00
	Approx., amount saved per month			
(i)	Rs. 25 or less		7	28.0
(ii)	Rs. 26—50		9	36.0
(iii)	Rs. 51 to 75		1	4.0
(iv)	Rs. 76—100		5	20.0
(v)	Rs. 101 and above		3	12.0
		Sub-total	25	100.0

families owed sums between 3001 to 4000; 13.05 per cent between 4001 to 5000; and only 7.24 per cent owed sums more than rupees 5000.

Regarding sources of debt it was found that contrary to the popular belief only 21.74 per cent families took loans from professional money lenders at 10 per cent rate of interest or more. A clear majority of 36.24

per cent sought recourse to friends and relations securing interest free loans in most cases. Another 21.74 per cent were indebted to their employers again on a reasonable terms. Some progressive families *i.e.*, 20.28 per cent had formed co-operative societies and got loans at low interest rate of 5 per cent.

In regard of saving habits our sample conformed to popular beliefs since only 21.74 per cent families reported regular monthly savings against 78.26 per cent having none. Table 3.5 shows that amongst the regular savers, a larger proportion saved, relatively speaking, lesser amounts per month. More specifically, 28 per cent saved rupees 25 or less per month and another 36 per cent reported monthly amounts between 26 and 50. There were 4 per cent in the range of 51 to 75; 20 per cent between 76 to 100 and only 12 per cent could save more than rupees 101 per month.

3.6 Housing, Access to Public Utilities and Environment

Although the very word "Slum" gives one a fair idea of housing, availability of public utilities and environmental conditions of the resident people, it was thought fit to collect empirical data pertaining to them for two specific reasons.

Firstly, it was on account of the high relatedness of the above stated factors to the physiological, mental and social health of individuals and secondly it provided us a reason for a systematic and detailed observation and understanding of home environment of our future partners in the field experiment.

The survey revealed that 69.56 per cent homes were over crowded having housing area of less than 250 square feet while the remaining 30.43 per cent families occupied area in the range of 251 to 500 square feet. Regarding type of housing, it was interesting to note that a majority dwelt in semi-pucca 47.82 per cent or pucca-20.50 per cent type of accommodation. Only 32.17 per cent families lived in kutcha houses.

Availability of protected water supply within a reasonable distance from residence is a luxury enjoyed by only some slum dwellers in Baroda city. Amongst the study families it was found that a large proportion *i.e.*, 43.47 per cent families had water tap within 24 ft. from their house; 26.95 per cent had between 25 to 49 ft., 10.43 per cent families had between 50 to 74 ft., 7.82 per cent had between 75 to 99 ft. and 11.30 per cent had it between 100 to 124 ft. However, it must be recorded that due to overall water shortage in the city since few years that study families got supply only twice during a day for half an hour each time. This produced considerable strain on the women. To a certain extent we too were constrained by the water timings while scheduling the various health interventions for children as well as mothers. Domestic electricity connections were taken by 56.52 per cent families while the remaining 43.47 per cent did without electricity in their homes.

The data on latrines, drainage facility and garbage disposal service, pass a sad commentary on the state of hygiene and sanitation. A whopping 95.65 per cent families had to use open grounds as latrines; (in absence of privately or publicly owned latrines) health hazards posed by which need no elaboration. Only 4.34 per cent families had privately owned but dry sanitation type (without water seal) of latrines. Drainage in the immediate surroundings was available to only 6.95 per cent families whereas 93.04 per cent families went without it. Similarly, whereas garbage disposal service from the municipal corporation was available to only 8.69 per cent while a majority *i.e.*, 91.30 per cent had to do without it.

Daily Diet Patterns and Percapita Intake of Essential Foods

Nutritional assessment of children and a follow-up health education to mothers was greatly enhanced by a diet survey. The exercise was meant to provide information about the types and amounts of foods consumed by target people. The findings were then compared against recommended nutritional standards to spot deficiencies of faulty practices, if any, for corrective education later.

Table 3.6A presents quantitative analysis of dietary patterns and is supplemented in its explanation by some additional observations for qualitative presentation.

Table 3.6B presents per capita consumption of essential foods matched against recommended dietary intakes for Indians as per ICMR (1981) report.

Several methods of diet surveys were considered for their virtual merits and demerits in the context of the given slum setting and resources at hand, both technical and financial. Finally, recall method of 48 hours was chosen for our purpose. The principle involved here is that the subject, or the home-maker in this case was asked to recall the types and amounts of food which had been eaten by the family during the past 48 hours. For assessment of quantities of food consumption the respondent was also asked to furnish data on monthly requirements of grains, pulses, vegetables, oils, sugar etc. Since the target families have extremely simple food habits, the respondents did not face much difficulty in recall. The investigators were indeed instructed clearly to inquire into this area after adequate

TABLE 3.6A: Daily Diet Patterns

	Class of Information	Distribution F	Distribution %
	Morning Tea		
(i)	No morning tea	18	15.66
(ii)	Only morning tea	47	40.86
(iii)	Roti with morning tea	33	28.69
(iv)	Bread or biscuits with morning tea	17	14.79
	Total	115	100.00
	Lunch		
(i)	Yes	115	100.00
(ii)	No	0	0.00
	Total	115	100.00
	Evening Tea		
(i)	No evening tea	89	77.39
(ii)	Only evening tea	26	22.61
(iii)	Snacks with evening tea	0	0.00
	Total	115	100.00
	Dinner		
(i)	Yes	115	100.00
(ii)	No	0	0.00
	Total	115	100.00

rapport establishment during the length of the interview.

Table 3.6A depicts some startling facts. All families have only two meals a day. Although there were wide variations in timings of the first and second meal, in most cases there was a long gap of about 8 to 10 hours in between. This runs counter to the medical advice of not keeping more than 4 hours gap between two consecutive meals and secondly that one should take three meals during a day.

Breakfast was dispensed with by 56.53 per cent families and only 43.47 per cent had it in form of left over 'roti' with tea-28.69 per cent or bread/biscuit with tea-14.78 per cent. A bulk *i.e.*, 40.86 per cent had only morning tea while 15.65 per cent had nothing at all.

Lunch and dinner were taken universally. During the recall of 48 hours food intake a general pattern emerged in which lunch consisted of *'roti'* with curried vegetable and dinner comprised either of *'khichadi'* or 'rice and dal' at times accompanied by a vegetable. Of the vegetables

TABLE 3.6B : Mean Intake of Essential Food Items Per Day

Food Item	ICMR (1981) recommended per capita daily Intake (I) (gms)	Daily Mean Intake			
		Per Capita (II)		Per consumption unit (III)	
		Mean (gms)	S.D. (gms)	Mean (gms)	S.D (gms)
Milk	175	52.36	18.67	63.66	18.67
Rice}	Cereals	200.67	7.76	243.41	7.76
Atta*}	= 500	235.25	8.89	261.45	8.89
Pulses	35	25.64	1.65	31.18	1.65
Vegetables	Roots: 55	102.71	4.63	130.64	4.53
	Leafy: 80				
	Others: 45				
	Total: 180				
Sugar	30	30.61	2.09	37.22	2.09
Oils/fats	35	24.22	1.40	29.45	1.40

* Wheat flour in most cases. Occasionally bajra and other varieties of cereals were reported.

reported commonest ones were potatoes, brinjals, cauliflower, tuwar (legume), tomatoes etc. The former two are relatively cheaper perennials while the latter were seasonal vegetables. Greens or leafy vegetables were conspicuous by their absence and same was true of milk products like curds or *'chaas'*. None reported *'salads'* and fruit. The reason for non-consumption of leafy vegetables usually given was that "on cooking they reduce in bulk and fall short". However on special occasions they do use fenugreek greens or *'Methi'* in combination with pulses or cereals like 'bajra' to make snacks. There was marginal reporting of non-vegetarian foods like mutton or eggs. Here, low consumption was more due to economic reasons than cultural factors.

Few families *i.e.*, 9.4 per cent with a little hesitation revealed that they have to beg every night for their dinner. As such they eat what they get.

Evening tea could be afforded by one 22.6 per cent and the rest 77.30 per cent did without it. None reported light snacks with evening tea.

Table 3.6B depicts nutritional gap at a glance with column I presenting ICMR (1981) recommendations for daily per capita food intake. While column II presents quantities consumed by a mean person in the community regardless of age, sex and type of work routine, column III gives a more objective view as it speaks of a standardized consumption unit in each household. For the present purposes, a standard person or consumer unit was defined by using Djurfeldt and Lindberg's method (explained in details under section 3.2 in this ch.)

It is clearly evident from Table 3.6B that except for milk and vegetables, daily food intake per consumption unit (refer column III) lies in close vicinity of specified quantities in column I while the data in col. II presenting non-converted per capita levels projects a falsified nutritional gap pertaining to cereals and pulses as well. Hence the importance of applying concept of consumption per household. The belief that the urban poor suffer a protein gap has been proven to be a myth by Parikh (1982).

Regarding milk consumption our experience during pilot testing needs to be mentioned. Unaware of existing reality, we had a direct question on daily milk consumption in terms of 'grams'. But on a number of occasions we got answers in terms of Rs. 1,2 or even 50 Paise etc. implying that they bought small quantities as and when required from vendors living in the neighbourhood. Unlike upper classes, they did not have a fixed delivery made to them everyday. Later during data collection, the investigators were instructed to modify their approach suitably in order to get realistic values.

In a study of Health status of 700 slum families of Baroda, Argade (1987) also reports a wide nutritional gap of milk and milk products. As the study does not present mean consumption values, a direct comparison with present data is not possible.

Regarding vegetables, it has already been reported earlier in this section, that their diet is grossly deficient of leafy vegetables since they were not mentioned at all during recall of 48 hours of food intake by any of the families. They exhibit greater preference for the cheaper potatoes, brinjals or seasonal vegetables which do not shrink in volume after cooking.

However, the overall picture seems to be less alarming when contrasted against data for urban Gujarat according to which 53 per cent households lie below recommended level—*Economic and Political Weekly* (1979). In absolute terms, there were, indeed several deficient areas and practices, which warranted corrective educational programme.

The on-going discussion of consumption levels of standardised units, per capita levels and ICMR recommendations would be incomplete without mentioning the well known and strong criticism levelled by Professor Sukhatme of the underlying methodology attempted by various authors. According to him, the recommended nutritional requirement is an average and not the minimum required for regular functioning of the metabolic system. Further, he says that the metabolic system of a body collapses when the calorie intake falls short of the minimum and not the average requirement. Therefore, use of average calorie requirement as the criterion for classifying a person as undernourished or poor can't be justified. This theory extenuates the nutritional status of study families to some extent.

3.7 Incidence of Pregnancy Wastage and Mortality of Underfives

Incidence of pregnancy wastage *viz.*, miscarriages, abortions or still births and mortality of underfives, particularly amongst infants are some of the most eloquent indicators of development (Perhaps that is why the statistical appendix attached to UNICEF Annual Report, 1984, lists the countries of the world not in the ascending order of their gross national products but in descending order of their I.M.R.). That is so because the statistics under discussion have as much to say about the quality of childrens' lives as about the numbers of their deaths.

Under the present study, we inquired into occurrence of any miscarriage, abortion or still-birth at any point in family history; age and sex of the child in case of death of an underfive and also the cause. Since precise data regarding cause of death was not available in all cases, the information has been excluded form tabular presentation.

Less than half *i.e.*, 43.47 per cent families exhibited a healthy trend

TABLE 3.7 : Incidence of Pregnancy Wastage and Underfives' Mortality

Variable	Distribution	
	F	%
Reported Pregnancy Wastage	17	14.78
Reported Underfives' Mortality	45	39.14
Dual Incidence of Pregnancy Wastage and Underfives' Mortality	3	2.60
Nil Incidence of Pregnancy Wastage and Underfives' Mortality.	50	43.48
Total	115	100.00
Age at death in case of Underfives only		
(i) 0-1 year	46	69.70
+		
(ii) 1-5 years	20	30.30
Sub-Total 66	100.00	
Sex of underfives who died		
(i) Male	38	57.58
(ii) Female	28	42.42
Sub-Total	66	100.00

with 'nil' incidence of pregnancy wastage or underfives' mortality. By implication, every second family had experienced loss of one kind or the other. More specifically, 14.78 per cent reported pregnancy wastage, 39.14 per cent reported underfives' mortality; and 2.60 per cent families reported mishaps of both types. Regarding age at death, it was found that of the total occurrence of 66 underfives' deaths, a majority *i.e.*, 69.70 per cent succumbed below one year while the rest 30.30 per cent died between one to five years. This clearly projects vulnerability of infants below one year. A reverse trend was observed regarding 'sex' of underfives who died. More male children *i.e.*, 57.58 per cent as compared to 42.42 per cent of female children lost their lives. As for causes of death, though precise data was not available in all cases, the commonest reasons given were diarrhoea, fever and mother's illness etc. Research studies in developing nations have shown diarrhoea and respiratory infections, mostly pneumonias to be killer childhood diseases ranking first and second respectively—UNICEF Annual Report (1984).

3.8 Utilization of Ante-natal, Natal, Post-natal and Family Planning Services

Utilization of services favourably affecting health of underfives comes as a natural sequel to the discussion of their quality of life (expressed by certain indicators) in the previous section. Developing Societies, usually exhibit low levels of utilization of health or other developmental service. (In overall terms, this was found true in present study also) This has often been attributed first, to paucity, of resources and second to lack of awareness amongst beneficiaries about services, it is also said that the poor do not value health as an asset and therefore, their efforts in maintaining it are at best half-hearted. What is not commonly known is the fact that the capacity of the poor to utilize services, despite awareness and access to them (services) is depressed due to poverty conditions. Chow (1984) puts this succintly in saying that persistent conditions of poverty produce certain incompetencies and a sense of deprivation which further debilitate the poor. Such a handicapped start in life reduces their abilities to benefit from available opportunities or make fullest use of developmental services and make attempts to lift themselves above the prevailing misery.

About the study sample Table 3.8 presents that only 4.34 per cent women had availed of regular ante-natal check up as against 93.91 per cent who had not; while 1.73 per cent were sterility or 'not applicable' cases. Here, regular periodicity was defined as at least two check-ups in each tri-mester. The primary aim of ante-natal care is to achieve at the end

TABLE 3.8: Utilization of Ante-natal, Natal, Post-natal and Family Planning Services

Variable		Distribution F	%
** Regular Periodic visits for ante-natal care and advice*			
(i)	Yes	5	4.34
(ii)	No	108	93.93
(iii)	N.A.	2	1.73
	Total	115	100.00
	Whether Vitamins and Iron supplements were taken		
(i)	Yes	74	64.36
(ii)	No	39	33.91
(iii)	N.A.	2	1.73
	Total	115	100.00
	Whether Tetanus Toxoid injection was taken		
(i)	Yes	59	51.30
(ii)	No	54	46.96
(iii)	N.A.	2	1.74
	Total	115	100.00
*** Place of delivery*			
(i)	Home (without trained birth attendants)	138	43.40
(ii)	Hospital	180	56.60
	Total	318	100.00
	Six week post-natal examination of mother and child		
(i)	Availed	9	7.83
(ii)	Not availed	104	90.44
(iii)	N.A.	2	1.73
	Total	155	100.00
	Post-natal Professional advice regarding		
(i)	Colostrum		
	Utilised	67	58.27
	Not Utilised	46	40.00
	N.A.	2	1.73
	Total	115	100.00
(ii)	Nutritious diet		
	Utilised	78	67.83
	Not Utilised	35	30.44
	N.A.	2	1.73
	Total	115	100.00

(iii)	Family Planning		
	Utilised	65	56.53
	Not Utilised	48	41.74
	N.A.	2	1.73
	Total	115	100.00
	Measures of contraception		
(i)	No permanent measure	48	41.74
(ii)	Permanent measure		
	Tubectomy	41	35.66
	Vasectomy	23	20.00
	Sterilisation by both spouses	1	0.87
(iii)	N.A.	2	1.73
	Total	115	100.00

* Periodic visits implied at least two check-ups during each trimester

** Response recorded for only last three children in each family.

of pregnancy a healthy mother and a healthy baby. Most women in the present study sought medical advice only in the last three months or the advanced stage of pregnancy. This perhaps explains why utilization levels of Iron supplements, Vitamins and Tetanus Toxoid were somewhat better. While 64.34 per cent had taken vitamins and Iron supplements, 33.91 per cent responded to negative and 1.73 per cent were sterile couples. Regarding Tetanus Toxoid injection 51.30 per cent responded in affirmative; 46.95 per cent in negative, the remaining 1.73 per cent being sterile.

Next aspect considered was that of trained attendance at delivery (a natal service). The women were asked to furnish data pertaining to last three or less (in case of lesser children) children born to them. Of the total such 318 births, 43.39 per cent were home deliveries *i.e.*, without trained attendance (they were also asked if any trained *dai* etc. was present at home delivery. All responded in negative) and 56.60 per cent were hospital deliveries where professional help was utilized which ensured delivery with minimum injury to the infant and mother; thorough asepsis; and competent expertise to deal with various natal complications Park and Park (1979: 426).

About customary six-week post-natal examination of mother and child, the figures once again are depressing. Only 7.82 per cent had consulted physicians within six-weeks of delivery and that too because the child developed some serious health problem. It is surprising that despite more than half the births having occurred at hospitals, 90.43 per cent women did not go back for post natal check up.

In Indian setting, colostrum or breast-secretion within 48 hours of childbirth is considered impure and discarded. On the brighter side, it was found that 58.26 per cent women had followed medical advice of giving colostrum to the new born child. Of the remaining women, 40 per cent discarded it (colostrum) while 1.73 per cent had no experience of child birth. Children deprived of colostrum are in effect deprived of protein rich nutrients and protective antibodies providing life-long immunity of certain types.

67.82 per cent women reported having adhered to professional advice regarding post-partum nutritious diet for health of mother and child. 30.43 per cent replied in negative and 1.73 per cent were childless.

Professional advice for spacing births or sterilisation was utilized by 56.52 per cent women while 41.73 per cent utilized neither of the two (services). 1.73 per cent did not need such advice. Further query into (permanent only) measures of contraception revealed that a large number *i.e.*, 41.73 per cent couples had not undergone either spouse sterilization. Tubectomy (Female sterilisation) was greatly favoured over vasectomy (Male sterilisation) the statistics being 35.66 per cent and 20.0 per cent respectively. This is despite the fact that vasectomy is much simpler an operation than tubectomy. Could the higher rate of female sterilisation vis-a-vis male sterilisation then be a pointer to low status of women? There was a unique couple or 0.86 per cent of the sample who reported sterilisation of both husband and wife.

TABLE 3.9 : Age at Weaning Practice

Weaning age in months		Distribution	
		F	%
(i)	4—6	12	10.44
(ii)	7—9	30	26.28
(iii)	10—14	52	45.16
(iv)	15—19	10	8.56
(v)	20—24	11	9.56
(vi)	25 and above	0	0.00
	Total	155	100.00

Mean age at weaning = 11.3 months
S.D. =2.3 months

Model class of weaning practice = 10 to 14 months.

Age at Weaning

The weaning period is the most crucial period in child development. But what does weaning mean? It means not sudden withdrawal of child from the breast. It is a gradual process starting around the age of 4 to 6 months because breast-milk alone is not sufficient to sustain growth beyond 6 months. It should be supplemented by suitable foods which are rich in nutrients and also easily digestible. In the Indian context soft cooked rice with dal, 'khichadi', rice water, boiled vegetables, half boiled egg, mashed banana, fruit juice, cow's milk etc. can be given.

If weaning is not carried out at the recommended age with recommended foods, the infant may fall prey to the vicious circle of mal-nutrition, infections and growth-faltering. In fact this is happening to millions of children in the world. The mal-nutritioned children contract diarrhoea and prolonged spells of growth faltering follow.

Of Indian poverty groups, it is believed that weaning is done most un-scientifically. Therefore, it was decided to collect facts at the local community level which could serve as apt illustrations during the health education programme later. Table 3.9 reveals grossly incorrect weaning practices amongst the study sample. Only 10.43 per cent could be credited for initiating weaning at the correct age group of 4 to 6 months. 26.28 per cent can be termed as 'moderately late starters' having begun weaning when the child was 7 to 9 months old. 45.16 per cent formed the modal class where the child was in the age group of 10-14 months when weaning began. Amongst the 'severely late starters' 8.69 per cent began weaning when the child was 15 to 19 months old; and another 9.56 per cent delayed weaning till the child was 20 to 24 months old.

Mean age at weaning was found to be quite high at 11.3 months with a standard deviation of 2.3 months.

The most popular weaning foods were 'rice'n dal' or *'khichadi'*. Many families give *'roti'* and *'dal'* or whatever is cooked for the family. Specially suitable weaning food was reported to be glucose biscuits (?). Few women prepared 'dal soup', 'rice-water', or fruit juice for infants. Top-milk *i.e.*, supplementary skimmed buffalo milk or cow's milk was given by only a small minority. One young mother had been giving 'Bournvita' to the infant at the time of data collection.

Motor and Mental Development Testing of Children between 0-30 months

Originally, under present study it was also intended to identify hidden disabilities amongst 0-30 month olds for organising appropriate health interventions towards improvement in their condition. Accordingly, Bailey's motor and mental development testing scale which has been standardised for Indian children by Dr. Pramila Phatak, Department of Child Development, Faculty of Home Science, M.S. University of Baroda was also included in the base-line survey. Prior to data collection, the investigators were sent for training in administration of the scale to Infant Testing Centre, Faculty of Home Science, M.S. University of Baroda. However, not a single case of disability amongst 0-30 months old children could be identified in the slum under study. This is understandable in the background knowledge that in a study of childhood disability conducted by Baroda Citizen's Council and UNICEF only 65 children in the said age group were identified from July 1983 to June 1986 in 325 slums under investigation. In other words, only 1 child from every fifth slum suffered such hidden disability. As such subsequent health interventions in our project got circumvented.

4

HEALTH AND GROWTH-MONITORING INTERVENTIONS

Affecting measurable (in statistical terms) improvement in health and growth of under-five slum children through professional social interventions was the ultimate goal set for the present experiment. This chapter illustrates impact of all health care and growth-monitoring activities denoted as input 'A' in introductory chapter one.

In the said context, researcher had postulated seven hypotheses as given in section 1.6.3. and the assessment of these based on Student's t-test would be presented serially. Two bar diagrams have been added to pictorially compare the treatment and control groups at pre- and post-intervention stages.

Thirdly, we include here results of multiple regression analysis between some relevant predictor variables like household size, mother's age, mother's education and per capita monthly income; and criteria variables like weight for height; haemoglobin status and nutritional status of the study children.

However, before we proceed with actual presentation of results, it is necessary to explain the following:

(i) Why monitor growth?
(ii) Modus-operandi for present study.
(iii) Rationale for selection of criteria indicators.
(iv) Important characteristics of Criteria indicators.

It may be recalled here that the concept of Growth Monitoring has been already presented in chapter one.

4.1 Why Monitor Growth?

First, the fact that mal-nutrition and resultant poor health in children remains invariably invisible till it attains dangerous proportions.

A detailed review of several hundred nutrition programmes conducted by the Harvard Institute for International Development (1981) concluded that:

> The Average moderately malnourished child in 6-24 months age range looks entirely normal but is too small for his or her age, has lowered resistance to infections and therefore easily succumbs to illness.
>
> The child receiving only 60 per cent of caloric requirement may give no outward sign of hunger beyond a frequent desire to breastfeed. In the Philippines study, 58 per cent of the mothers of second and third degree malnutritioned children said their babies were growing and developing well.

Secondly, ignorance of required nutrients leads to improper diet causing malnutrition. Studies undertaken in several countries, including India have shown that more than half of all cases of malnutrition are to be found in households where there is no absolute shortage of food. The reason why available food is not given to a malnourished child is usually that the mother does not know that her child is becoming undernourished and also that a child has special nutritional needs. And in many cases, the child's own appetite is depressed-often by the same illness which is causing malnutrition.

Thirdly, the noteworthy fact that growth-monitoring interventions are extremely cost-effective even when applied to large populations on a mass scale. The appropriate technology for it are Road-to-Health cards (available for 50 p. each) described later in section 4.4.3.

Lastly, and most importantly, concept of growth-monitoring is revolutionary in the sense that it essentially involves the mother in the child health concerns.

Mother: the one person who loves and cares for the child the most. If and when the mother is empowered with the following simple message:

— Weight gain from one month to the next is good.
— Weight constant is not good;
— Weight loss is a serious danger signal.

She (the mother) can do the most to prevent or correct any undesirable trends.

In conclusion, we quote UNICEF (1987) —

> As a technique, growth-monitoring can give an early warning of growth-faltering. As a process, it can be a channel for new information on growth promotion. And as a focal point for child health care, it can help shift the emphasis from professionals to parents, from clinics to communities, from dependence to empowerment. And in so doing, it can help to build genuine primary health care.

4.2 Modus-operandi for the Present Study

True to all that has been said above, during the present field-experiment we came across several mothers oblivious of their child's endangered health. Invariably the mother felt her child was well because he or she was 'easy to look after' and/or 'liked to eat' etc. The mother could hardly be labelled as ignorant or negligent because the child seldom presented any outwardly signs of malnutrition like skin lesions, a swollen belly, light coloured hair, signs of apathy or illness (cold, cough, fever, diarrhoea) etc. It was only when we had the initial assessment of haemoglobin level done and each child plotted on Road-to-Health cards, for his or her 'weight for age' parameter, did it become apparent that only a small minority of study children possessed good health.

Now, explaining growth charts and monitoring results can be done either in a group or through one-to-one counselling or discussion with the mother of her respective child's weight gain or weight loss and the concomitant interpretations were usually carried out on-the-spot *i.e.*, the matter was taken up immediately after anthropometric measurements. This was possible due to the valuable assistance provided by the CHV and the field work students. At times, few mothers did leave before the discussion of results (owing to other pressing engagements) but later they invariably contacted the researcher on their own to inquire about the same.

Growth monitoring through the group medium was also quite effective. The mothers listened in rapt attention when we cited live examples from their own environment and of children known to them. The women were encouraged and guided to reflect on questions like:

What could be the cause?

What needs to be done now?
Could it have been prevented?
Who should do what?
Special situations of children of working or widowed mothers.
Food fads of children.
Economics of nutrition etc.

It turned out to be one of the areas in which maximum number of women participated and made the discussions lively. Besides, the women were both positive and respectful to others in their deliberations. On our part we were careful that mothers of malnutritioned children were not singled out in an awkward manner and embarrassed. Also, the mothers who had tried to practice recommended feeding were called upon to share their experiences of whether they faced any problems; how did they solve the problems; and what modifications they would like to suggest etc.

It was also required to monitor vitamin and iron supplements to each child as prescribed in order to ensure correct use without a break or discontinuation of the drug altogether. Although this was the assigned responsibility of the CHV, initially the researcher also went around the community to gain first hand knowledge of the field level realities. In most cases, there were no serious difficulties. Occasionally mothers complained that the children made a fuss about taking the medicine. Mothers of very small children found it genuinely difficult to administer the tonics even in powdered form with sugar. Such children were supplied with paediatric syrups in lieu of tablets. At times when the child was down with an infection, the mother stopped giving the tablet. We decided to respect her judgement at that instant but advised that the treatment be resumed when the child recovered health.

4.3 Selection of Criteria Indicators

According to Rao (1986: 77) selection of indicators should depend on the following:

(i) It should be reliable and available on regular basis from the same set of populations collected under comparable conditions;
(ii) It should be simple enough to collect, analyse and interpret even at the peripheral and immediate level; and
(iii) Above all the indicator should bear a theoretical relationship with the condition which is being measured or monitored.

In other words, availability, simplicity, reliability, comparability, and relevance are the essential characteristics of a good indicator. Under the present study, all selected indicators with the exception of 'incidence of morbidity' to some extent not only had the above characteristics for a good measure but these could be defined un-ambiguously, in clear terms, too. Description of these indicators now follow.

4.4 Characteristics of Criteria Indicators

4.4.1 *Weight for Height*

Although, in general terms, 'weight for age' (in case of children) is a sound measure of health and nutrition, in India its interpretation is accompanied by serious flaws as the true age of the child is not known many a time.

In an attempt to find a truly age dependent index, Rao and Singh (1970) compared heights and weights of apparently normal children with no signs of mal-nutrition and coming from low socio-economic families in Hyderabad city, India. They found that ratio Weight/Height^2 x 100 was remarkably constant over the age range of 1 to 5 years and was the same for males and females. Their mean value for normal children was 0.15 and for those with signs of Protein Energy Malnutrition (PEM) it ranged between 0.12 and 0.14.

For the present study, we adopted the above stated standards as the children belonged to low socio-economic groups. Secondly, height and weight data could be reliably collected by our community health volunteer under proper guidance.

4.4.2 *Haemoglobin Estimation*

It is the most important laboratory test that is carried out in health and nutritional studies. Park and Park (1985: 110) state that haemoglobin is a useful index of overall state of nutrition irrespective of its significance in anaemia.

In our study, we secured the necessary expertise and logistics support from S.S.G. Hospital, Baroda, for collection and analysis of samples.

For interpretation, we used WHO standard regarding haemoglobin content in under-five children *i.e.*, 11.0 gm/dl. as the cut off point to set apart the healthy from the weak.

4.4.3 *Nutritional Status*

At the outset, it needs to be clarified that although haemoglobin and 'Weight for Height' are themselves good indicators of nutritional status, for the present purposes, the criterion variable 'nutritional status' exclusively refers to the readings from Road-to-Health cards used for growth-monitoring. The cards obtained from S.S.G. Hospital, Baroda had two sets of weight for age graphs: separate for infants under one year and for those between one to five years of age (please refer appendix). For grading nutritional status we used a classification by UNICEF and Ghose (1976) as per below:

Area between Curves	Per-centile of median weight	Nutritional Status.
top-most and one below	80%	Satisfactory
second and third from top	80-71%	Ist degree of malnutrition
third and fourth from top	70-61%	2nd degree of malnutrition
fourth and fifth from top	Under 60 per cent	3rd degree of malnutrition

The card 'inter-alia' helps early and easy (at-a-glance) detection of growth faltering so that mothers could be advised and alerted in time.

4.4.4 *Incidence of Morbidity*

Recording of morbidity or sickness in a community study is always a ticklish issue. That is so because reporting of sickness is a highly subjective matter. Besides, there usually remain gaps in definitions of illnesses and interpretations of probe questions amongst all concerned *viz.*, investigators, respondents, subjects (whose health is under study) and professionals.

According to Pathak (1985) who conducted a study of perceived morbidity and utilisation of health services in slums of Nagpur city and 43 villages in Saoner taluka, medically defined illnesses are 2.24 and 3.6 times higher than perceived illnesses amongst infants and 1-5 year old children respectively.

Therefore, for the present study we decided to have our own method of data keeping of morbidity. The trained community health volunteer visited door-to-door and inquired from mother's whether their children under the project had a spell of diarrhoea, skin disease, cough and cold, low grade fever, high grade fever, measles, chicken pox or any other ailment during the past week. The CHV passed on the data to the researcher the very next day for information and necessary action. Such type of record was maintained from Ist March to 31st August 1987 i.e. the period in which all health care and growth-monitoring interventions were carried out.

4.5 Results based on Hypothesis Testing

Assessment of the seven hypotheses related to health and growth-monitoring interventions is discussed hereafter.

4.5.1 *Hypothesis 1: The mean value of Weight/Height² x100 index of growth in treatment group children would show increase after the experiment vis-a-vis the mean value before.*

To test the above hypothesis, pre-intervention mean weight/height ^{2}x 100 value recorded in Feb '87 was compared and subjected to paired samples' t-test alongwith the post-intervention mean value recorded in Aug '87. Table 4.1 furnishes the details. It can be seen that the two said values were. .1295 and .1411 respectively and the increase was statistically highly significant at p=.000 level; degrees of freedom being 29. Hence the hypothesis is accepted.

TABLE 4.1: t-test Analysis: Pre-Post Means of Wt./Ht² x 100 Index in Treatment Group

Paired Samples:

V_{13} — Weight by Height² x 100: Feb. '87 data.

V_{16}- Weight by Height² x 100: Aug. '87 data.

No of cases: 30

Degrees of Freedom: 29

Variable	Mean	S.D.	Correlation	t-Value	2-Tail Value
V_{13}	.1299	.009			
V_{16}	.1411	.008	.853	-13.88	.000*

* Extremely Significant at 0% level.

As stated earlier in section 4.4.1 the mean value for normal Indian children from low socio-economic groups is 0.15. This implies that the children were in very poor health before the experiment and although there was significant improvement in their growth after six months of intervention they (children) could not still reach the normal level. However they did come quite close to the normal value.

Hypothesis 2: The mean value of Weight/Height² x 100 index of growth in treatment group children vis-a-vis the control group children would be higher after the experiment.

To test the above hypothesis, it was first necessary to establish that the two groups were initially well matched and highly comparable on the criterion of weight/height^2 x 100. This was done by subjecting the pre-intervention mean values to independent samples t-test as shown in table 4.2A. The table shows that the mean values of .1295 and .1301 in treatment and control group respectively were statistically not different at P=.820, degrees of freedom being 53. In other words the two groups based on the criterion in question were much alike before the experiment. This very fact has been pictorially presented in Fig. 4.1.

TABLE 4.2A: t-test Analysis: Pre-Intervention Means of Wt./Ht.^{2} x 100 Index in Treatment and Control Groups. n of Treatment Group = 30; n of Control Groups = 25

				Pooled Variance Estimate		
Group	Mean	S.D.	F Value	t-Value	d.f. Prob	Tail Value
Treatment	.1295	.009				
			1.12	-.23	53	.820*
Control	.1301	.009				

* Not Significant at 5% level.

TABLE 4.2B : t-test Analysis: Post-Intervention Means of Wt./Ht. 2*100 Index in Treatment and Control Group

				Pooled Variance Estimate		
Group	Mean	S.D.	F Value	t-Value	d.f Prob	2-Tail Value
Treatment	.1411	.008				
			1.05	4.19	53	.000*
Control	.1320	.008				

* Extremely significant at 0 % level.

Next we sought to establish that after the interventions the mean values in both groups stood statistically different. Table 4.2B depicts post-intervention mean values of weight/height^2 x 100 as .1411 and .1320 in treatment and control group respectively. The mean difference of .0091 was found to be statistically highly different at p= .000. Hence, hypothesis 2 is retained.

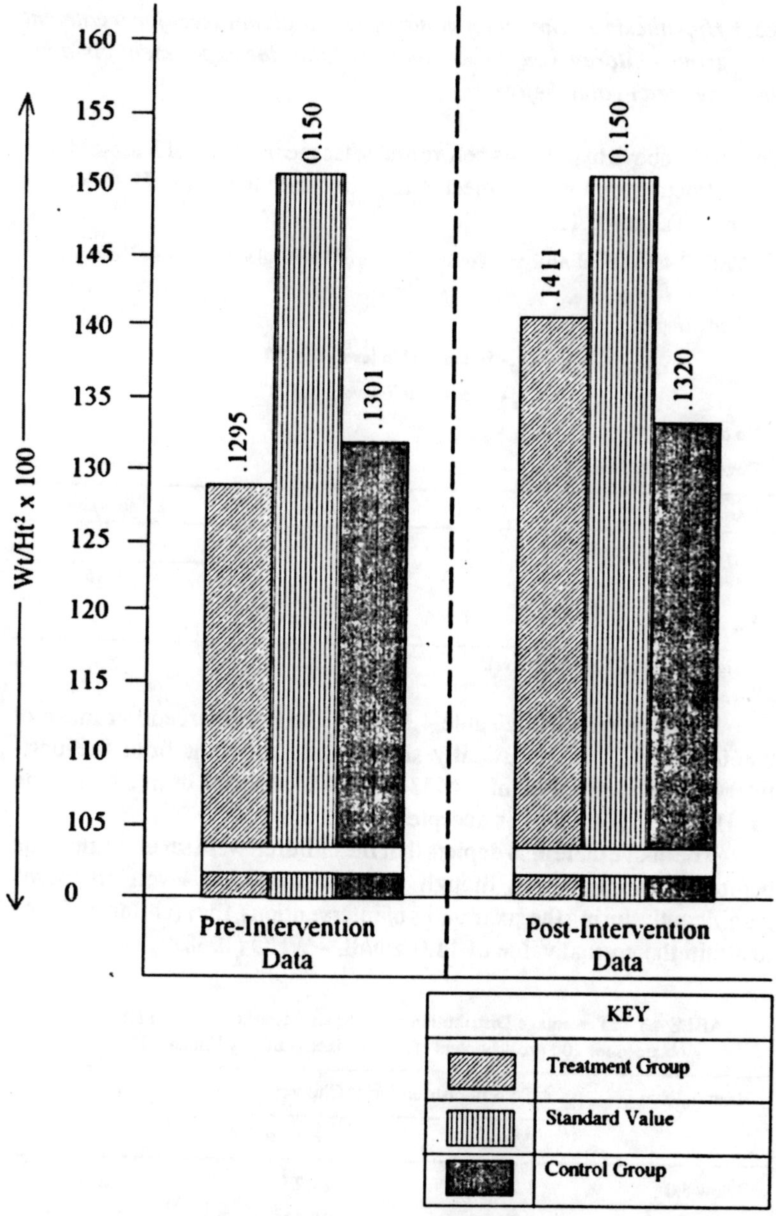

SCALE : 0.1 Cm = .001 Measure of Wt/Ht² x 100

Fig. 4.1 : Pre and Post Intervention Weight-for-Height Measure in Treatment and Control Groups

4.5.3 *Hypothesis 3: The mean value of haemoglobin level for treatment group children would show increase after the experiment vis-a-vis the mean value before.*

To test the above hypothesis before and after mean values of haemoglobin in treatment group were subjected to paired samples t-test. Detailed are given in Table 4.3.1.

TABLE 4.3.1 : t-test Analysis: Pre-Post Means of Haemoglobin Status in Treatment Group.

Paired Samples:

V_{17} - Haemoglobin level; Feb '87.

V_{18} - Haemoglobin level; Aug '87.

No of Cases: 30

Degrees of Freedom: 29

Variable	Mean	S.D.	Correlation	t-value	2 Tail Value
V_{17}	8.8600	1.364			
			.587	– 2.58	0.15*
V_{18}	9.4433	1.366			

* Significant at 1.5 per cent level.

It can be seen from Table 4.3.1 that the pre-intervention mean of 8.8600 gm/dl. was statistically significantly different from the post-intervention mean value of 9.4433 at p= .015; degrees of freedom being 29. Hence, hypothesis 3 is accepted.

The above table also depicts that the children were severely anaemic before intervention and though their haemoglobin levels improved significantly during the six months of interventions, they (children) failed to attain the normal value of 11.0 gm/dl. - WHO (1968).

TABLE 4.3.2 : Percentage Distribution of Children According to Mean Hb levels as obtained for 200 pre-schoolers of Rural Hissar-study by Kakkar (1987).

Haemoglobin	Percent distribution of Children		Total
	Male	Female	
Below 5.0	1.27	1.27	2.53
5.00 to 6.9	8.86	10.13	18.99
7.00 to 8.9	30.38	26.58	56.96
9.00 to 11.0	13.92	7.60	21.52

Kakkar (1987) in a study on nutritional status of pre-school children in rural Hissar (N = 200) also found very low levels of haemoglobin amongst study children Table 4.3.2 reproduced from the study above may be referred. Similarly, Gopaldas (1986) also found low haemoglobin level amongst under-fives *i.e.*, of the order of 7.4 gm/dl. These studies have been quoted to bring out the fact that anaemic condition amongst pre-school Indian children from low socio-economic strata seems to be an ubiquitous phenomenon.

However, since our intervention could successfully achieve positive change in the intended direction, it may be concluded that such interventions for extended period could contribute immensely towards health of under-fives.

4.5.4 *Hypothesis 4: The mean value of haemoglobin level for treatment group children vis-a-vis control group would be higher after the experiment.*

To verify the above hypothesis, it was first necessary to establish that the two groups were initially well matched and highly comparable on the criterion on haemoglobin status. This has been done by subjecting the pre-intervention mean values to independent samples t-test as shown in Table 4.4A. The table shows that the mean haemoglobin values of 8.8600 and 8.7160 in treatment and control groups respectively were statistically not different at p= .680; degrees of freedom being 53. In other words, the two groups based on the said criterion were much alike before the experiment. This very fact has been presented pictorially in Fig. 4.2.

TABLE 4.4A: t-test Analysis: Pre-Intervention Means of Haemoglobin Status in Treatment and Control Groups

n of Treatment Group = 30

n of Control Group = 25

Group	Mean gms/dl	S.D. gms/dl	F Value	Pooled Variance Estimate t-value	d.f.	2-Tail Value
Treatment	8.8600	1.360				
			1.35	.42	53	.680*
Control	8.7160	1.174				

* Not Significant at 5% level.

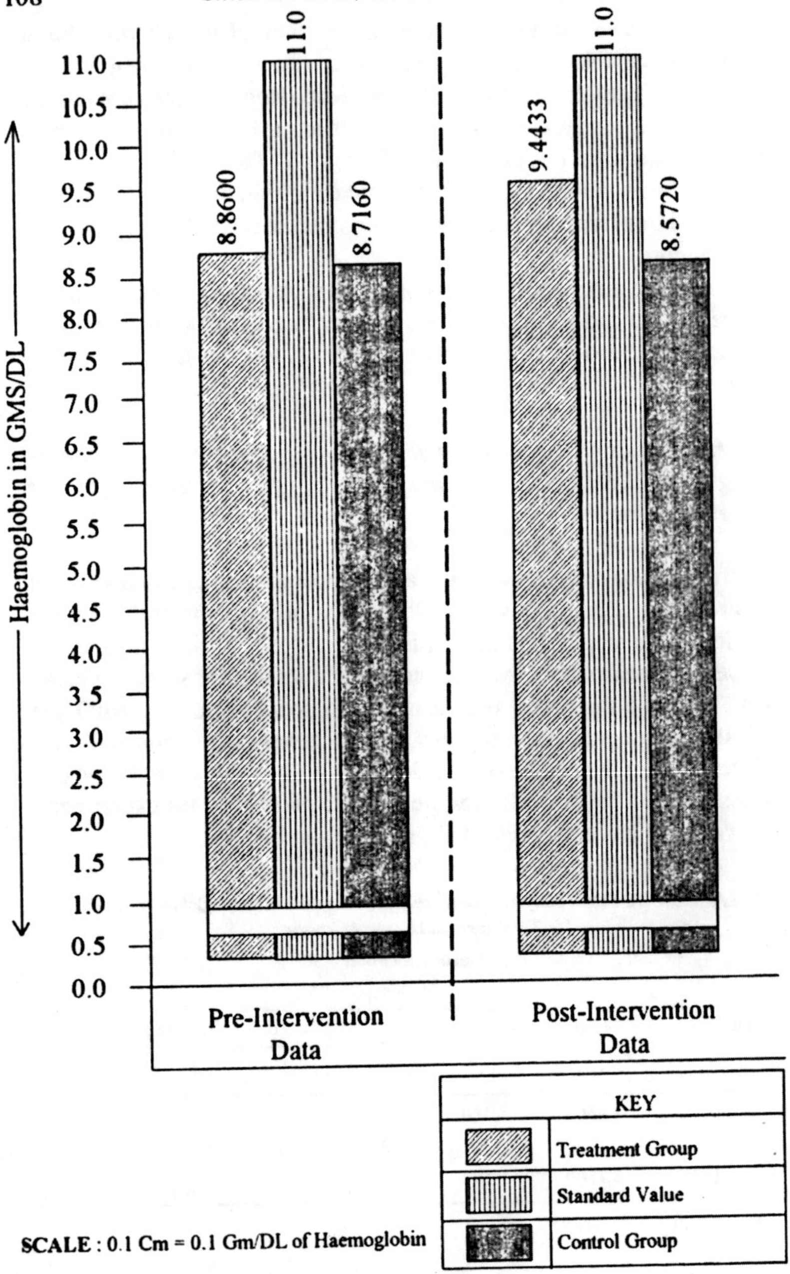

SCALE : 0.1 Cm = 0.1 Gm/DL of Haemoglobin

Fig. 4.2 : Pre and Post Intervention Haemoglobin Levels in Treatment and Control Groups

TABLE 4.4B: t-test Analysis: Post-Intervention Means of Haemoglobin Status in Treatment and Control Groups

Group	Mean gms/dl	S.D. gms/dl	F Value	Pooled Variance Estimate t-value	d.f	2 Tail Value
Treatment	9.4433	1.366				
			1.38	2.52	53	0.15*
Control	8.5720	1.1623				

* Significant at 1.5 per cent level.

Next we sought to establish that after the intervention the mean values in both groups stood statistically different. Table 4.4B depicts post-intervention mean values of 9.4433 and 8.5720 in treatment and control group respectively to be statistically different at $p = .015$ level of significance; degrees of freedom being 53. As the F-value was 1.38 pooled variance estimate was made. Hence hypothesis 4 is accepted.

4.5.5 *Hypothesis 5: The mean value of nutritional status for treatment group children would show increase after the experiment vis-a-vis the mean value before.*

To test the above hypothesis before and after mean values of nutritional status in treatment group were subjected to paired samples t-test. Details given in Table 4.5

TABLE 4.5 : t-test Analysis: Pre-post Means of Nutritional Status in Treatment Group

Paired Samples:

V_{19} - Nutritional Status Feb. '87

V_{22} - Nutritional Status Aug. '87

No. of Cases: 30

Degrees of Freedom: 29

Variable	Mean	S.D.	Correlation	t-value	2 Tail P value
V_{19}	3.0333	.718			
			.477	5.19	.000 **
V_{22}	2.4000	.563			

** Extremely Significant at 0 per cent level.

* Variable code:

1 = Satisfactory nutritional status.
2 = 1st degree of mal-nutrition.

3 = 2nd degree of mal-nutrition.
4 = 3rd degree of mal-nutrition.
5 = 4th degree of mal-nutrition.

It can be seen from Table 4.5 that the pre-intervention mean (please refer variable code in this Table) of 3.0333 was statistically significantly different from the post-intervention mean value of 2.4000. Hence hypothesis 5 is accepted.

Despite the fact that the nutritional status of treatment children improved significantly, Table 4.5 illustrates that they (children) merely moved from 2nd degree of mal-nutrition somewhere close to 1st degree of mal-nutrition only. This implies that more inputs or perhaps the same inputs for a longer duration are required to raise the children's nutritional status to a satisfactory level.

In a study conducted in Central India, Gopaldas (1986) showed that 75 per cent of children in the age group 0-6 years suffered from second and third degree mal-nutrition. Similarly, Kakkar (1987) in an earlier mentioned study found that only 18 per cent children had normal or satisfactory level of nutrition. The remaining were distributed as: 38 per cent in grade I; 31 per cent in grade II; 9 per cent in grade III and 4 per cent in grade IV of mal-nutrition. These findings reflect that the children in our study conformed to the prevailing trends of mal-nutrition amongst under-fives children.

4.5.6 *Hypothesis 6: The mean value of nutritional status for treatment group children vis-a-vis control group would be higher after the experiment.*

To verify the above hypothesis it was first necessary to establish that the two groups were initially well matched and highly comparable on the criterion of nutritional status. This was done by subjecting the pre-intervention mean values to independent samples t-test as shown in Table 4.6A. The table shows that the mean nutrition status (coded as shown in the table) of 3.0333 and 3.1402 in treatment and control groups respectively were statistically not different at p=.708; degrees of freedom being 53. In other words, the two groups based on the said criterion were much alike before the experiment.

TABLE 4.6A: t-test Analysis: Pre-Intervention Means of Nutritional Status in Treatment and control groups

n of Treatment Group = 30

n of Control Group = 25

				Pooled Variance Estimate		
Group	Mean	S.D.	F Value	t-Value	d.f.	2 Tail-P-Value
Treatment	3.0333	.718				
			1.24	.65	53	.708*
Control	3.1402	.695				

* Not Significant at 5 per cent level.

TABLE 4.6B: t-test Analysis: Post-Intervention Means of Nutritional Status in Treatment and Control Groups

	*			Pooled Variance Estimate		
Group	Mean	S.D.	F Value	t-Value	d.f.	2 Tail P Value
Treatment	2.4000	.563	1.46	2.58	53	0.36**
Control	2.9802	.688				

** Significant at 3.6 per cent level.

* Variable code:

1 = Satisfactory nutritional status
2 = 1st degree of mal-nutrition.
3 = 2nd degree of mal-nutrition.
4 = 3rd degree of mal-nutrition.
5 = 4th degree of mal-nutrition.

Next, we sought to establish that after intervention, the mean values in both groups stood statistically different. Table 4.6B depicts post-intervention mean values of 2.4000 and 2.9802 in treatment and control groups respectively to be statistically different at p= .036 level of significance; degrees of freedom being 53. As the F-Value was 1.46 pooled variance estimate was made.

Hence hypothesis 6 is accepted

4.5.7 *Hypothesis 7: The mean reported incidence of each of the eight morbidity conditions viz-diarrhoea, vomitting, measles, chicken pox, skin diseases, high grade fevers, low grade fevers, coughs and colds (there was 'nil' response for the ninth category—any other) under observation during the intervention period in treatment group would be lower than the corresponding values for control group at the end of the experiment.*

The above stated hypothesis virtually consists of eight parts *i.e.*, the eight morbidity conditions as mentioned for which the treatment and control groups were observed throughout the six months of intervention. As per the hypothesis we were interested in only the post intervention situation of both groups. Accordingly, the mean occurrence of each condition in the last month of intervention *i.e.*, Aug. '87 in both groups were subjected to independent samples t-test. Details are presented in tables 4.7.1, 4.7.2, 4.7.3, 4.7.4, 4.7.5, 4.7.6, 4.7.7, 4.7.8 interpretations of which are taken up serially now.

4.5.7.1 *Post-intervention Reporting of Diarrhoea*

TABLE 4.7.1 : t-test Analysis: Post-Intervention Reported Incidence of Diarrhoea in Treatment and Control Groups

n of Treatment Group = 30

n of Control Group = 25

			F	Pooled Variance Estimate		
Group	Mean	S.D.	Value	t-Value	d.f.	2 Tail P Value
Treatment	1.5333	1.456				
			1.47	2.12	53	0.39*
Control	.7600	1.200				

* Significant at 3.9 per cent level.

Table 4.7.1 shows that in treatment group mean reporting of diarrhoea was 1.5333 as against .7600 in control group *i.e.*, the mean reporting was higher in treatment group vis-a-vis control group—a situation diametrically opposite to the stated hypothesis. Besides, the difference of means was statistically significant at p= .039; degrees of freedom being 53. How do we account for this? How is it that the treatment group children after under going a rigorous health care intervention package experienced higher morbidity than the control group children who received no health care at all? Since the treatment group children had shown significant improvement on all the major health indicators there was no reason to accept a proposition that our health care had nil or in fact, detrimental impact. Since the final outcome in some other morbidity conditions like measles, low grade fevers and coughs 'n cold were similar, the situation was rather baffling initially, to say the least.

An exhaustive search of factors responsible for the unexpected curious trends, led to the following possibilities:

(i) As stated earlier, may be there were lacunae in data collection itself *i.e.*, the community health volunteer did not work sincerely or the discharge of supervisory role by the researcher was unsatisfactory etc. In other words, due to some such reasons, the data on hand had low/no validity. However, the researcher does not believe that any of the above were true. We have enough confidence in the work of CHV and also the supervisory instrument set up.

(ii) Having ruled out the above possibility, we suggest here what we believe to be one of the true causative factors.

It may be recalled that our research design incorporated a regular, continuous and welfare-oriented contact between the researcher and the treatment group mothers through the apparata of growth-monitoring discussions and health education sessions. On the other hand, the researcher maintained only an occasional contact with the control group mothers, say during anthropometric measurements, clinical examinations, haemoglobin testing or chance meetings on her (researcher's) various community visits. As such it is quite likely that while the treatment group mothers developed genuine interest in the project and co-operated by sincerely reporting morbidity as per their perceptions; the control group mothers felt rebuffed and were careless to report. Therefore, it should be noted that higher reporting of morbidity by treatment group mothers does not necessary mean that the actual morbidity levels in their children were higher, due to the reason just discussed.

(iii) The second important causative factor seems to be a direct out come of our health education intervention. The treatment group mothers were not only imparted knowledge of common childhood diseases, how to care for and manage the child during each specific illness but were also stimulated to develop right kind of attitudes towards 'health'. Attempts were made to make them more health conscious; to perceive health as a valuable asset; to believe in the old cliche-'prevention is better than cure'; and to realise the importance of early detection and timely treatment of a disease for its control. These inputs in treatment mothers led them to report more frequently.

The situation in this project seems similar to the falsified increase in incidence of Diabetes Mellitus, Cancer, heart conditions etc. in recent years as compared to past. Higher reporting of morbidity does not necessarily mean rise in actual incidence but suggests that people are better aware and report sickness in early stages.

4.5.7.2 *Post-intervention Reporting of Vomitting*

TABLE 4.7.2 : t-test Analysis: Post-Intervention Reported Incidence of Vomitting in Treatment and Control Groups

Group	Mean	S.D.	F Value	Pooled Variance Estimate t-Value	d.f.	2 Tail P-Value
Treatment n=30	.5333	.571				
			1.01	1.12	53	.267*
Control n=25	.3600	.569				

* Not Significant at 5 per cent level.

Table 4.7.2 shows that in treatment group mean reporting in Aug. '87 was .5333 as against .3600 in control group i.e. mean reporting in treatment group was slightly higher vis-a-vis control group—a situation defying the stated hypothesis. However, the difference of means was not wide as to make it significant at $p < .05$ (as shown in Table 4.7.2). In order to explain this un-expected finding we offer the reasons described in detail in section 4.5.7.1 as (i), (ii), (iii).

4.5.7.3 ***Post-intervention Reporting of Measles***

TABLE 4.7.3 : t-test Analysis: Post-Intervention Reported Incidence of Measles in Treatment and Control Groups

Group	Mean	S.D.	F Value	Separate Variance Estimate t-Value	d.f.	2-tail P-Value
Treatment n=30	.1000	.305				
			2.33	.87	50.40	.386*
Control n = 25	.0400	.200				

* Not Significant at 5 per cent level.

Once again mean reporting of measles in treatment group was slightly higher as compared to mean value of control group; the precise figures being .1000 and .0400 respectively. However, the difference was not so wide as to make it significant at $p < .05$ as shown in Table 4.7.3. Here sinçe the F-value was 2.33 separate variance estimate was made.

To explain this unexpected result, we attribute the same reason discussed at length in section 4.5.7.1 as (i), (ii), and (iii).

4.5.7.4 *Post-intervention Reporting of Chicken Pox*

TABLE 4.7.4 : t-test Analysis: Post-Intervention Reported Incidence of Chicken Pox in Treatment and Control Groups

Group	Mean	S.D.	Computer Warning
Treatment n=30	.0333	.183	No Variance for Independent Sample t-test.
Control n=25	.0000	.000	(One or more samples has no variance)

Table 4.7.4 clearly depicts that there was only a marginal difference between the mean reporting in treatment group: .0333 and mean value of control group:- .0000 the variance was so negligible that the computer issued a warning: No variance for Independent Samples t-test (one or more samples has no variance).

It must be conceded here that there was no need to inquire about incidence of chicken pox in the month of August as the ailment is usually seasonal, occurring mainly in summers. Perhaps this explains 'nil' or low reporting in both groups.

4.5.7.5 *Post-intervention Reporting of Skin Diseases*

TABLE 4.7.5 : t-test Analysis: Post-Intervention Reported Incidence of Skin Diseases in Treatment and Control Groups

				Pooled Variance Estimate		
Group	Mean	S.D.	F Value	t-Value	d.f.	2 Tail P-Value
Treatment n=30	.5333	1.570				
			1.41	.67	53	.504*
Control n=25	.8000	1.323				

* Not Significant at 5% level.

This was first instance, where as expected, we found that mean reporting in control group was higher as compared to mean value of treatment group as obtained in Aug. '87. However, the difference was not large enough, so that the hypothesis 7 could be retained at p < .05 level of significance as shown in table 4.7.5. As the F-value was 1.41 pooled Variance estimate was made.

The hypothesis in this case is clearly rejected.

4.5.7.6 *Post-intervention Reporting of High Grade Fevers*

TABLE 4.7.6 : t-text Analysis Post-Intervention Reported Incidence of High Grade Fevers in Treatment and Control Groups

				Separate Variance Estimate		
Group	Mean	S.D.	F Value	t Value	d.f.	2 Tail P Value
Treatment n = 30	.3333	.711				
			2.66	.60	49.01	.533*
Control n = 25	.2400	.436				

* Not Significant at 5% level.

Contrary to hypothesis 7, the mean reporting of high grade fevers in treatment group vis-a-vis control group was higher in Aug. '87; the exact figures being .3333 and .2400 respectively. The difference of means was however, not so large as to make it significant at p < .05 as shown in Table 4.7.6. As the F-value in this case was 2.66 separate variance estimate was made. To explain this unexpected result, we put forth the same submissions, presented in detail in section 4.5.7.1 as (i), (ii) and (iii).

4.5.7.7 *Post-intervention Reporting of Low Grade Fevers*

TABLE 4.7.7 : t-test Analysis: Post-Intervention Reported Incidence of Low Grade Fevers in Treatment and Control Groups

				Pooled Variance Estimate		
Group	Mean	S.D.	F Value	t-Value	d.f.	2 Tail P Value
Treatment n = 30	2.0667	1.530				
			1.59	3.25	53	.002*
Control n = 25	.8400	1.214				

* Extremely Significant at .2 per cent level.

Table 4.7.7 clearly depicts that mean reporting of 2.0667 in treatment group was considerably higher as compared to mean reporting of .8400.

The difference was highly significant at p=.002; degrees of freedom being 53. As the F-value in this case was 1.59 pooled variance estimate was made as shown in the table.

Once again the reality situation is diametrically opposite to the stated hypothesis and we attribute it to the same causative factors, discussed at length in section 4.5.7.1 as (i), (ii) and (iii).

4.5.7.8 *Post-intervention Reporting of Coughs and Colds.*

Table: 4.7.8 t-test Analysis: Post-Intervention Reported Incidence of Coughs and Colds in Treatment and Control Groups.

				Pooled Variance Estimate		
Group	Mean	S.D.	F Value	t-value	d.f.	2 Tail-P-Value
Treatment n=30	3.2000	2.140				
			1.02	2.27	53	0.028*
Control n=25	1.8800	2.166				

* Significant at 2.8 per cent level.

Once again, Table 4.7.8 clearly depicts a trend contrary to the stated *i.e.*, incidence in treatment group was considerably higher vis-a-vis control group. The difference of means was large enough to be significant at p = .028; degrees of freedom being 53. Since the F-value was 1.02, pooled variance estimate was made as shown in the table.

Here too, we explain the un-expected results by putting forth the same reason-(i), (ii) and (iii) discussed in section 4.5.7.1 at length.

4.6 Results of Correlation and Multiple Regression Analysis

Multiple regression analysis is one the most important tools which makes possible the study of direction and magnitude of effects of more than one independent variables on one dependent variable. That precisely served our purpose as we were interested in studying the correlation between our major dependent criterion variables and some independent predictor variables like household size, mother's age, mother's education and per capita monthly income as also the extent of variance that each of the latter variables could produce with regard to the former.

Understanding of the nature and quantum of these relationships empowers us with the tested knowledge towards improving practice of, more specifically in this case, how predictor variables could be manipulated in designing further interventions for promoting health of underfives from low socio-economic groups. The following three sub-sections present findings related to weight for height measure, haemoglobin and nutritional status.

4.6.1 *Correlation and Multiple Regression between Criterion Variable Weight/Height² x 100 and Predictor Variables as listed below: Household size, Mother's Age, Mother's Education and Per Capita Monthly Income.*

Table 4.8.1 shows that of all the predictor variables in the equation, V_{28} *i.e.*, mother's education had the strongest positive correlation of .284 with the dependent variable weight/height² x 100.

Multiple regression analysis reveals that of all the variables in equation only V_{28} *i.e.* mother's education is positively and significantly related to weight for height measure. The level of significance is quite high *i.e.*, .0079 and the variance produced is 13.66 per cent (value of R square). According to Reid (1981) in social work research models that can explain 15 per cent of variance are considered good enough. Therefore, in our present model variance of 13.66 per cent caused by mother's education level is quite close to 'good enough'. It should also be noted that partial

TABLE 4.8.1: Correlation and Multiple Regression between Criterion Variable V_{36} *i.e.* Wt/Ht.² x 100 and Predictor Variable as listed below

Variable	Label	Mean	Standard Deviation
V_{25}	House hold size	5.527	1.289
V_{28}	Mother's Education	1.709*	.994
V_{32}	Per Capita M. Income	111.382	57.448
V_{33}	Mother's age	25.418	3.895

N of Cases = 55

Correlation:

	V_{25}	V_{28}	V_{32}	V_{33}	V_{36}
V_{25}	1.000	-.052	-.271	.671	.099
V_{28}	-.052	1.000	.316	-.174	.284
V_{32}	-.271	.316	1.000	-.133	.002
V_{33}	.671	-.174	-.133	1.000	.001
V_{36}	.099	.284	.002	.001	1.000

Multiple Regression:

Method: Enter

EQ 1 V_{36}

(Wt./Ht.^{2} x 100)

Variables in Equation

Variable	B	SEB	T	Sig-T
V_{33}	1.549570E	3.12368E-04	.495	.6229
V_{32}	– 1.45208E-05	1.71742E-05	–.846	.4019
V_{27}	1.256286E-04	2.08354E-03	.060	.9522
V_{28}	2.629236E-03	9.49840E-04	2.768	.0079
V_{25}	– 3.77625E-04	1.05575E-03	– .358	.7221
(Constant)	2.311634E-03	6.61375E-03	.350	.7282

Multiple R .36954

R Square .13655 or 13.66 per cent

Adjusted R square .04844

Standard Error 6.373105E-03

Variable Codes·

* 1 = Illiterate

2 = 1 to 5 years of formal education

3 = 6 to 9 years of formal education

4 = 10 to 12 years of formal education

regression co-efficient or Beta weight for V_{28} *i.e.* mother's education was .002629 indicating that when all the other independent variables were held constant or controlled, V_{28} added considerable variance.

How does the above finding add to social work knowledge? In a poor country like India where per capita incomes are amongst few of the lowest in the world; households usually large; and the trend of early marriage quite common, it is certainly an encouraging revelation. It is encouraging because our intervention model has clearly demonstrated that income, household size and mother's age had only a negligible impact on the dependent variable in question. The high, positive correlation with mother's education emphasises importance of raising women's education in the society for improving health standards of underfives.

4.6.2 *Correlation and Multiple Regression between Criterion Variable-Haemoglobin Status and Predictor Variables as listed below:*

Household size, Mother's Age, Mother's Education and Per Capita Monthly Income

TABLE 4.8.2 : Correlation and Multiple Regression between Criterion Variable V_{37} *i.e.*, Haemoglobin and Predictor Variables as listed below:

Variable	Label	Mean	Standard Deviation
V_{25}	House-hold size	5.527	1.289
V_{28}	Mother's Education	1.709 *	.994
V_{32}	Per Capita M. Income	111.382	57.448
V_{33}	Mother's Age	25.418	3.895
	N of cases = 55		

Correlation

	V_{25}	V_{28}	V_{32}	V_{33}	V_{37}
V_{25}	1.000	–.052	–.271	.671	–.117
V_{28}	–.052	1.000	.316	–.174	.383
V_{32}	–.271	.316	1.000	–.133	.161
V_{33}	.671	–.174	–.133	1.000	–.128
V_{37}	.099	.284	.002	.001	1.000

Multiple Regression:

Method: Enter

EQ 1 : V_{37} (Haemoglobin)

Variables in Equation

Variable	B	SEB	T	Sig-T
V_{33}	–5.18621E-03	.05275	.098	.9221
V_{32}	8.390816E-04	2.90044E-03	.289	.7736
V_{27}	–.25256	.35188	–.718	.4763
V_{28}	.40769	.16041	2.542	.0143
V_{25}	–.02690	.17830	–.151	.8807
(Constant	.07921	1.11696	.070	.9445

Multiple R .40614

R Square .16495 or 16.495 per cent

Adjusted R square .07974

Standard Error 1.07632

Variable Code

*1 = Illiterate

2 = 1 to 5 years of formal education

3 = 6 to 9 years of formal education

4 = 10 to 12 years of formal education

Table 4.8.2 reveals that house-hold size and mother's age were negatively correlated with haemoglobin status implying that smaller households, and low age of mothers produce positive effect on haemoglobin increase in the children. However, the correlations were low *i.e.* –.117 and –.128 for V_{25} and V_{33} respectively and made no statistically significant impact. Per Capita monthly income was positively related; implying that higher the income, higher the increase in haemoglobin level. This indeed is self-explanatory in the sense that persons with higher incomes had higher purchasing power for adequate and nutritious food so necessary to raise an individual's haemoglobin level. Here too, the relationship was not statistically significant. Education level of mother, was once again found to add considerable variance (with B = .40769) to the dependent variable when other predictor variables were held constant. The positive impact made by this variable was also significant at .014 level; implying that increase in mother's education leads to definite and significant increase in haemoglobin level (in the present intervention model). Value of R square; was also quite high *i.e.*, 16.495 per cent which according to Reid W.J. (1981) was better than 'good enough' level of 15 per cent Variance.

4.6.3 *Correlation and Multiple Regression between Criterion Variable Nutritional Status and Predictor Variables as listed below: Household Size, Mother's Age, Mother's education and Per Capita Monthly Income.*

TABLE 4.8.3: Correlation and Multiple Regression between Criterion Variable V_{38} *i.e.* Nutritional Status and Predictor Variance as listed below:

Variable	Label	Mean	Standard Deviation
V_{25}	Household size	5.527	1.289
V_{28}	Mother's Education	1.709 *	.994
V_{32}	Per Capita M. Income	111.382	57.448
V_{33}	Mother's Age	25.418	3.895
	N of Cases = 55		

Correlation

	V_{25}	V_{28}	V_{32}	V_{33}	V_{38}
V_{25}	1.000	–.052	–.271	.671	.075
V_{28}	–.052	1.000	.316	–.174	.295
V_{32}	–.271	.316	1.000	–.133	.070
V_{33}	.671	–.176	–.133	1.000	–.087
V_{38}	.075	.295	.070	–.087	1.000

Multiple Regression:

Method: Enter

EQ 1 : V_{38}

(Nutritional Status)

Variable in Equation

Variable	B	SE B	T	Sig T
V_{33}	-.03391	.03774	-.899	.3733
V_{32}	2.022273E-05	2.07494E-03	.010	.9923
V_{28}	.21707	.11476	1.892	.0505
V_{25}	.01895	.12755	.820	.4165
(Constant	.01895	.79906	.024	.9812

Multiple R .34241

R Square .11724 or 11.72 per cent

Adjusted R square .02717

Standard Error .76998

Variable Code

*1 = Illiterate

2 = 1 to 5 years of formal education

3 = 6 to 9 years of formal education

4 = 10 to 12 years of formal education

Table 4.8.3 shows that of all the predictor variables only 'mother's age' bore a negative correlation with the dependent variable, namely, nutritional status. This implied that younger mothers had healthier children. However, the correlation matrix had low value of only –.087. From the remaining independent variables mother's education had the strongest positive correlation of .295 indicating that better educated mothers achieved higher nutritional status for their respective children. Multiple regression analysis further confirmed these findings. The relationship between mother's education and nutritional status of the child was statistically significant at $p = .05$ level. The variance produced or the R^2 value was 11.72 per cent which is rather satisfactory. Partial regression coefficient or Beta weight for V_{28} *i.e.*, mother's education was found to be .21707. Once again, present intervention model has suggested that by upgrading mother's education, it is possible to improve health of under-fives.

5

HEALTH EDUCATION INTERVENTION

Formulating a 'situation-practical' health education programme; conducting it on field; and evaluating its impact were some of the major goals of the field-experiment. While the operational definition, objectives and procedures of health education interventions have already been presented in chapter one under sub-section 1.6.6.2, 1.5.2 and 1.6.6.3 respectively; at this juncture we need to focus on two inter-related concerns, namely :

(i) How were the individual sessions conducted 'on field' and what were the exact inputs?
(ii) To what extent were the programme objectives achieved?

For an orderly presentation, discussions on (i) and (ii) above, have been consigned into two separate sections of this chapter as per below:

Section 5.1: Covering Content and Methodology of Individual Sessions.
Section 5.2: Reporting Impact of the Programme on Target Mothers.

However, before we proceed further, it is necessary first to give a brief account of the 'Basic Premises' on which the present HEP was founded as well as the theoretical principles of Health Education used by us at the implementation level.

Basic Premises

For a while, consider the following facts:

Indian women, generally speaking are frail persons having to undergo multiple pregnancies. They usually suffer from deficiencies of minerals and vitamins as well. Such women give birth to weak and 'at risk' off springs and high underfives' mortality ensues.

Woman, is also the chief person who cooks for the family and looks after all—young or old. As such, needless to say that it would mean a significant social investment if the woman is taught about basic facts of health care; functions of different foods; concepts of a balanced meal and the scientific methods of cooking so that the nutrients are conserved and not lost in the process.

Next, even if sound food and health habits are practiced one could fall sick due to a hoard of other reasons. The home-maker should therefore, know how to care for and manage the sick. She needs to be liberated of her superstitious ways affecting health and well-being of all. Further, she must be made aware of various preventive and curative health services, especially those available in her neighbourhood and she should also be made to feel inclined to utilise them.

And above all, she must learn to perceive health as a valuable asset and develop more positive attitudes towards herself and womanhood as a whole.

Thus, in view of the pivotal role of woman in Indian households, it is plain obvious that health education interventions for women possess a vast potential of raising health standards in the society. In recognition of this fact several state and voluntary agencies have incorporated HEPs for women as integral part of their health services. By the same token, the present interventive research would have been incomplete and in-effectual to an extent in the absence of an HEP.

Principles of Health Education

Of the immense literature available on principles and techniques of health education what resembles closest to Social Work methods in general and the present research model in particular is presented here. Once again, we quote Wilson (1948) for the Six Commandments of Successful Health Teaching listed as per below:

1. Consider individual differences.
2. Discourage self-diagnosis and self-medication.
3. Avoid embarrassing pupils.
4. Adapt teaching to pupils' interests, needs and capacities.
5. Base teaching on real life problems and real people.
6. Use a variety of teaching methods and finally—Actions speak Louder Than Words

SECTION 5.1

PRESENTS CONTENT AND METHODOLOGY OF HEALTH EDUCATION SESSIONS

A chronological account of the fifteen health education sessions conducted by us comprises this section. The style of reporting is necessarily of a 'summary type' highlighting only the most relevant features from our field notes. But we wish to place on record our strong belief that each and every moment spent by us with the target group contributed towards informal education of either. There were several inadvertent gains accruing from 'the fall-out process' of the programme. The most significant one being that the target mothers underwent a dramatic change in their personalities. From the stereotype of illiterate, under-priviledged and shy women they emerged as bold, relatively well aware and intellectually curious individuals in their own right. Most of our guest speakers were highly impressed by their keen interest in the programme and the quality of questions raised by them. To add further, a local, voluntary, womens' welfare agency after conducting community awareness programmes on 'Legal rights of women' in several slum locations of Baroda including Pensionpura acknowledged the superiority of our target group in terms of their 'participativeness and general smartness'.

With this short preamble, contents and methodology pertaining to each individual session of the health education programme now follow.

Session I

Date - 24-7-87

Time - 3.00 to 4.30 pm

Objectives:
(i) To orient the participants to the goals, subject matter content, duration, and methodology of implementing the health education programme.
(ii) To state the general rules of the programme; explain what benefits the women could derive as also the way in which they could contribute to make the programme successful.
(iii) Through media of games make target women aware of the importance of health for the mother and child.

Media Used:
(i) Group Discussions
(ii) Educative Games.

Process and Observation: It was the very first session. Kanuben, the CHV had informed the target women twice in advance about arriving at the Balwadi by 3.00 p.m. However, the researcher had to go door to door alongwith Kanuben to gather the women. Most of the women brought their small children along. Few older children came on their own as they were much curious to know why the women were called by us. Since the Balwadi area was rather small, probably less than 50 square feet, presence of children created lot of disturbance. Kanuben, aided by few volunteers was partially successful in making the children quiet.

At the outset, the women were told that approximately 15 such sessions would be held in which through different media of teaching like lectures, role play, story telling, film show etc. they would be educated about health and nutrition care of their underfive children. It was also emphasized that we would much prefer it to be a two-way process of exchange of ideas and clarification of doubts. The women should feel free to tell us if they felt that our theory was wrong. The smiles and noddings from the women were indicative of their approval.

The incentives to attend the programme were stated as below:

(i) Women attending 13 or more sessions would receive Ist Prize.
(ii) Women attending 11 or 12 sessions would receive IInd Prize.
(iii) Women attending 9 or 10 sessions would receive IIIrd Prize.
(iv) All women attending more than 9 sessions would receive a certificate in Child Health Education from Fatehgunj Samaj Kalyan Kendra (FSKK), an urban community development agency of Faculty of Social Work, M.S. University of Baroda.
(v) There would be few additional prizes awarded for their attentiveness and performance in health quiz games.

The women heard us attentively. Few asked about the utility of the said certificates. The example of Kanuben was given. The other women too could get similar jobs with relative ease if they earned their certificates.

In the latter half of the session a simple game was conducted which covered the following three aspects.

(i) Nutritious fruit for underfives.
(ii) Importance of family planning and spacing.
(iii) Weaning age.

(i) Nutritious Fruit for Underfives

Slips of papers depicting pictures of four fruit namely, Banana, Apple, Chikku and Grapes were distributed to the women and they were asked to tick mark the one fruit which according to them was the most suitable for their underfives. When the papers were collected, we scored them. Most women had voted for apple. In the discussion that followed they said apple was the best firstly because children liked it the most and secondly, because it was an expensive fruit and therefore, more health-giving. When we told them that the correct answer in this case was Banana, few of them protested that banana caused coughs and colds. Researcher was aware of this lay belief and she clarified the matter to them in the same lay language that banana would cause cold if the child drank water immediately after having it. The aim was to avoid a controversy in the very first session.

(ii) Importance of Family Planning and Spacing

Two charts were made for the purpose. The first one pictorially presented that proper spacing between the children led to a happy mother and healthy children. The second chart showed that less difference betweer children resulted in unhealthy children and an unhappy mother. The women began to identify their ownselves with the first or the second case. The researcher told them that their own situations could not be altered now but this knowledge gain would empower them to help their friends and relatives.

(iii) Weaning Age

Slips of papers containing four to five numbers were distributed to the women and they were asked to encircle one of them at which (month) weaning should start. Actually, many of them knew the correct answers that it should be done at four or five months of the child's age. On being asked whether they had practiced what they knew, most replied in negative and laughed. Few said by way of explanation, that they did not know all this when they were young mothers and few others said that their mothers-in-law did not allow them to do so.

> *Evaluation:* Fourteen women participated today. The general response to the games was good. During discussion, only three women spoke freely. Others were shy and special efforts were needed to enhance their participation.

Session-II

Date : 31-7-87
Time : 2.30 To 4.30 p.m.

Objectives: (i) Recapitulation of the previous session.
(ii) To give a talk on 'Balanced Meal' emphasizing importance of Iron, Calcium, Vitamin A and water.

Media Used (i) Group discussion.
(ii) Lecture with the aid of posters and chart.

Note: Originally we had planned for a pre-intervention 'health quiz' but since the women were not willing, the exercise was dropped.

Process and Observations: We began with the feed back of the previous session. Initially, the women were surprised that we asked them what they had learnt in the previous session. Gradually they warmed up and most of them were able to give correct answers, possibly because the coverage was not heavy and they were familiar with the subject. Their ability in answering correctly boosted their self-confidence and as a result they became more vocal.

In the latter part of the session talk on concept of a balanced meal was first taken up. They were told about the functions of nutrients like iron, calcium, vitamin A and water; sources of these; and deficiency diseases caused by inadequate consumption of the same.

Evaluation: The women listened attentively. Even though the terms were given in Gujrati , initially, they found the subject matter a bit difficult to comprehend. However, repetition by us seemed to be helpful to them. Some women got up and left the session for a while to attend to important domestic duties. This caused much disturbance and it was decided to counsel the women (not to do so) individually in their homes and not in the group itself. Neeruben, the adult education teacher of the slum area. took down notes entirely on her own initiative. At the end of the session we asked her whether she would like to present her notes further enriched by her own knowledge and experience to the rest of the group. Neeruben gladly accepted the responsibility.

Session-III

Date : 7-8-87
Time : 2.30 To 4.30 p.m.

Objectives: (i) Recapitulation of the previous lesson by Neeruben.
(ii) To continue the talk on 'balanced meal' by emphasizing importance of proteins, vitamins and fats.

Media Used (i) Paper presentation by volunteer from the Group.
(ii) Group discussion.

Process and Observations: The session started late by 45 minutes. This happened due to lashing rains in the area that day and the fact that women wanted to wash their large utensils (used on festive occasions) with the nature's bounty of rain water.

As decided, Neeruben presented her paper first. It was a brief paper but contained all the essential information; alongwith her own experience.

Later the researcher continued her talk on vitamins B, C, D, fats, proteins. In simple language they were told about the functions of these nutrients, their food sources and the diseases resulting from their deficiency.

Evaluation: This time we had erred in not using pictorial material for the talk—the participants looked confused. It was decided to make more charts for use in the next session on the same topic and to end that session with a quiz game which would help towards re-inforcement of the previous lessons.

Session-IV

Date : 14-8-87
Time : 2.30 To 4.30 p.m.

Objectives: (i) Consolidate teachings on the concept of 'balanced meal'.
(ii) Conduct a quiz Game.

Media Used (i) Display of charts.
(ii) A Quiz Game.

Process and Observations: Today only 10 women came. This happened because it was the ration collection day and the other women had not finished their purchases. The lesson learnt by us was that it was necessary to inquire about the suitableness of the date and time of the next session at the end of every session. We could not have a fixed time table as is possible in formal institutions of learning.

At the beginning, for about twenty minutes we displayed the charts containing illustrations of different foods, their sources and functions. We also told them that they should have a good look at the charts because after a while the charts would be removed and a quiz game on the same topic be conducted. The women were excited about the game and studied the charts carefully.

Conduct of Quiz Game

The women were made to sit according to their serial number in the attendance sheet. Then we told them that there were 13 questions in the quiz and the rules of the game were stated as follows:

(i) Each lady would be asked one question. She would be awarded 10 marks for right answers and zero for an incorrect answer.
(ii) In case the question was not answered or it was incorrectly answered it would be passed on to the lady immediately next and so on till the correct answer was given. Whosoever gave the right answer for a 'passed' question would be awarded 5 marks.

The result of the quiz game was as follows

S.No	Participant	Marks obtained
1.	RJ	10 + 10 = 20
2.	KP	10 + 5 + 5 + 10 = 30
3.	KT	10 + 10 = 20
4.	SG	10 + 10 = 20
5.	JL	05 + 10 = 15
6.	SN	05 + 10 =15
7.	MN	10 + 10 = 20
8.	SB	10
9.	NM	10
10.	ST	0

Quiz Question with Correct Answers

Q. 1. What are the common sources of Proteins?

Ans. Milk, curds, eggs, dried beans, peas, groundnut and other nuts, pulses, whole grains preferably sprouted.

Q. 2. What are the common sources of the vitamin A?

Ans. Butter, Ghee, Eggs, Carrots, Papaya, Mango, all leafy vegetables.

Q. 3. Which disease is caused due to deficiency of vitamin A?

Ans. Night blindness.

Q. 4. What are the sources of Vitamin B?

Ans. Sprouted grains, Whole Grains, milk, fermented foods like 'dhokala', 'idli' and 'dosa'.

Q. 5. What are the sources of vitamin C?

Ans. Lime, Amla, Guava, Tomatoes, Oranges and Grapes.

Q. 6. Which common disease is caused due to deficiency of vitamin-C?

Ans. Common cold.

Q. 7. What is the cheapest source of vitamin D?

Ans. Sunlight.

Q. 8. What is the most important function of vitamin D?

Ans. Aids in formation of healthy bones.

Q. 9. Which common and cheaply available fruit is a good source of calcium?

Ans. Banana.

Q. 10. What is the important function of calcium?

Ans. Aids in formation of healthy teeth and bones.

Q. 11. What are the important sources of Iron?

Ans. Jaggery, green vegetables, dates, channa.

Q. 12. What disease is caused by deficiency of Iron?

Ans. Anaemia.

Q. 13. How many grams of iron should there be in one deciliter of blood?

Ans. 11 grams.

Evaluation: The quiz game was very well received by the participants. As the result shows the learning by the group in this areas was fairly satisfactory considering that this was an entirely new subject for them.

Session-V

Date : 19-8-87
Time : 1.30 To 3.30 p.m.

Objective: (i) To impart knowledge of pre-natal and post-natal care.

Media Used (i) Talk by an expert *i.e.*, a Gynaecologist.

Process and Observation: Dr. (Miss) Trusha Zikare was invited. She was told in advance about the research project and background level of the participants and that she should deliver a talk on Pre-natal and Post-natal care.

The women came in time and in full strength. The contents of the expert's talk can be summarised as follows:

(i) Pre-natal Care

It was emphasized that as soon as a woman realises that she is pregnant she should immediately see a qualified doctor and not feel shy or hesitant. The pregnant mother should take a balanced diet and include cheap but nutritious items like bananas, jaggery, chana (Bengal gram) and whole grains preferably sprouted, in her meals. The pregnant woman should continue her household work as before. During rest and sleep time she should lie on the left side so that the embryo inside is provided with more blood. Tetanus Toxiod injections should be taken in the seventh, eighth and ninth month of pregnancy. It provided protection against Tetanus to the mother and child. Iron and calcium supplement tablets should be taken as per medical advice.

(ii) Post-natal Care

It is very important to remain in touch with the doctor after delivery also so that unnecessary infections can be avoided and correct advice received for subsequent immunization of the child as well as family planning.

(iii) There should be no discrimination between boys and girls.

Evaluation: After the talk, the doctor held a question answer session with the women on allied subjects of nutritive foods, weaning age, attitudes to family planning etc. She was much surprised to receive correct answers to all her questions. She was also impressed by their disciplined and yet active participation. The expert's comments were shared with the women to encourage them further. The women then took initiative in seeking advice on some of their problems regarding menstruation etc. We were fully satisfied today that our efforts were well directed.

Session-VI

Date : 21-8-87
Time : 2.30 To 4.30 p.m.

Objective: To emphasize upon the target women the importance of personal hygiene; in particular about cleanliness of nails, teeth and hands.

Media Used
(i) A skit by community children.
(ii) Group discussion.

Preparatory Work:
(i) Suitable modification of dialogues to Indianise the skit taken from (Teaching Health Education in the elementary School' by Wantz (1967).
(ii) Translation of the skit into Gujarati language.
(iii) Assigning the task of getting the skit ready to the field work students.
(iv) Preparation of masks for the children so that it becomes easy to identify the characters played by them in skit.

The Skit

Title: Dangerous Germs.
Skit Objectives:
(i) The skit brings out that some diseases are caused by micro-organisms.
(ii) Washing hands removes disease carrying micro organisms.

Materials Required

(i) Masks to specify germs; the skin cells; the portion of the body attacked by germs; water and paste; soap and water.

Moderator : This is a story of three germs named Pinku, Rinku and Tinku which attack the body of Bharat, a small sweet boy and try to make him sick. What we now present is a meeting between the three germs, who are good friends, always in search of a host.

Pinku : I am the most dangerous germ and can affect teeth

very badly. I like to cause tooth decay and can make Bharat cry with pain.

Rinku : Just this much? You don't know how dangerous I am! I shall enter in Bharat's nails and through his food enter into the mouth and meet you there. Then we shall work together to make him sick.

Tinku : I shall join you in a slightly different way. When Bharat comes to the park to play I shall just stick to his hands and through food enter the mouth.

All the three laugh together—

Ha! Ha! Ha!

All The Three together : This way we shall help our friend Disease to spread in Bharat's body and later attack his family members and neighbours.

(Scene II : Bharat wakes up in the morning.)

Mother : Bharat, get up! Brush your teeth and come for breakfast.

Bharat : I am very hungry. Nothing is wrong with my teeth. They are bright and white and do not need brushing!

Mother : No, no! Bharat, you must brush twice a day. I won't allow you to eat without brushing. When you eat, food particles get stuck on the teeth and germs can grow there (Bharat begins to brush his teeth)

Pinku : Oh-my God! What is this on me! My whole body is hurt and I am being thrown away.

Water & Paste : Cry for help. No one will help you!

Pinku : Help! Rinku, Tinku, Help! (No response)

(Scene III : After breakfast Bharat is getting ready for school)

Mother : Check whether your nails are properly cut or not-otherwise your teacher will scold you.

Bharat : Why should she scold? I won't cut them now, I am getting late.

Mother : Do cut them and remove dust particles settled underneath.

(Mother cuts the nails and cleans them).

Rinku : Hey! Someone is pulling me out of my place. Help me! (No response)

Scene : After School, Bharat played in the park and is back home.

Tinku : Hello! I am Tinku the germ and I like to make people sick.

Moderator : Lakshmi, Bharat's sister enters the room.

Lakshmi : Bharat, see What I brought for you?

Tinku : (Jumps up and down) I am now on Lakshmi's hand and I would like to make her sick too.

Skin Cells : Go away! You are very bad!

Tinku : I will make her sick. Ha! Ha! Ha!

Mother : Bharat, Laxmi! be sure that you wash your hands before you eat.

Lakshmi & Bharat : But our hands are not dirty!

Mother : But you might be having germs on your hands which are too small to be seen. But they are quite powerful to make you sick.

Lakshmi & Bharat : Alright mother.

Tinku : Help, Help! there is water and soap on me.

Soap & Water : We will kill you here and now. We won't let you make people sick.
(Tinku Cries ....)

Evaluation : The skit was very much appreciated by all. After complimenting the artistes we had a follow up discussion with women to assess how far our objective was served. It was encouraging to know that women not only understood the direct message of the skit but that they also grasped the indirect message about the responsibility of mother in ensuring cleanliness of the child.

Session-VII

Date : 26-8-87

Time : 2.30 To 4.00 p.m.

Objective : To impart knowledge of usual season of occurrence, common symptoms, complications and harmful effects, management and prevention of common childhood diseases, namely, Tetanus, Scabies and Diarrhoea.

Media Used : (i) Story-telling with the aid of flip charts.
(ii) Follow-up discussion

Note: 1. Illustrative flip charts with captions in Gujarati language were obtained from Sarabhai Science Centre, Ahmedabad.

2. A copy of one such story on Diarrhoea is attached as Appendix 'C'.

Process and Observation: The topic for coverage today was introduced and the women were told that we needed one volunteer from the group to conduct the session. The women looked somewhat baffled but when they were told that we had illustrative stories which the volunteer could read out they were satisfied. Neeruben was selected by the group to read out the stories.

Neeruben presented the stories in a humourous way and at the same time conveying the exact meaning. Some of the characters of the stories could be identified with few of the group members or their friends and that's how humour began. Few additional points which were not covered in the story were covered by the person in charge.

Evaluation : Story-telling medium was very much enjoyed by the women. Follow-up discussion revealed that the medium also provided much clarity of the subject. Participants were very happy on being told that a similar session would be held next week.

Session-VIII

Date : 2-9-87
Time : 2.30 To 4.00 p.m.

Objective : To impart knowledge of usal seasons of occurrence, common symptoms, complications and harmful effects, management and prevention of common childhood diseases, namely, Chicken Pox, Measles and Anaemia.

Media Used : (i) Story-telling with the aid of flip charts.
(ii) Follow-up discussion

Note : 1. Illustrative flip charts with captions in Gujarati language were obtained from Sarabhai Science Centre, Ahmedabad.

Process and Observations: The group members had brought few of their friends along, perhaps due to the success of the previous session. We said that we should have a different volunteer today. The group assigned the responsibility to our CHV, Kanuben. For Kanuben it was the first occasion to read out to a group from a formal platform but she did a good job of it.

As in the previous session. Follow-up discussion revealed that learning by the group was also of a high standard.

Evaluation : The interest generated by story-telling techniques could be gauged by the fact that group members brought their friends along for the session and also when they requested to have more stories in addition to the ones planned for the day. To honour the participants' request stories of Malaria and Pneumonia also presented.

Session-IX

Date : 4-9-87

Time : 2.30 To 4.30 p.m.

Objective : To emphasize significance and importance of spacing children and family planning.

Media Used : (i) Story-telling session by a worker from Kashiben Gordhandas Patel Children's Hospital, Karelibaugh, Vadodara.

(ii) Follow-up discussion.

Note : The guest speaker brought along her own illustrative material of flip charts.

Process and Observation: The session today was conducted by an experienced person and this was reflected in her ability to carry out ensuing discussion from the story-session. The story, in a nutshell was as follows:

Two ladies who were good friends were shown to visit a rural primary health centre together for advice on family planning. A public health nurse explains to them the advantages of using Copper-T and gives instructions about the same. One lady follows the advice and gets a Copper-T inserted by the qualified doctor and is able to plan her family. This results in a healthy and happy family.

On the other hand her friend did not heed the advice or rather was discouraged by the mother-in-law about it. The result was a poor and unhealthy family.

The guest speaker included in her presentation certain questions for women which were directed to help the latter in developing positive attitudes towards female children, the women themselves as well as family planning. The women participated actively and teased each other about related issues.

Evaluation: As in the past two sessions, the story techniques aided by flip charts was very well received and seemed to be impactful too.

Session-X

Date : 9-9-1987
Time : 2.30 To 4.30 p.m.

Objective : (i) Discuss reasons for utilization and non-utilization of health services.
(ii) Discussion on availability of health services in neighbourhood and at city level.
(iii) Discuss major social problems in India.

Medium Used : Free response of participants on any idea or theme presented by researcher.

Process and Observation: As the subject today was familiar to participants the emphasis was on getting maximum contribution from them during discussions. The women were told that one by one topics would be mentioned and they should speak on it whatever comes to their mind first *i.e.*, it was intended to be a kind of a buzz session, which was subsequently supplemented by researcher. The responses of the women were as follows:

(i) Health Services in Neighbourhood and Around

Weekly immunization clinics run by Baroda Municipal Corporation, neighbourhood anganwadis under ICDS project, health services provided by S.S.G. Hospital, Community outreach services and hospital based services of Kashiben Children's Hospital. Health Services under U.C.D, Baroda Project, missionaries' health services at Lady Pillar Hospital, made up the consolidated list. What different services are available at each of the above centres were also discussed.

(ii) Reasons for Non-utilization of Health Services

The participants said that they prefer private clinics to S.S.G. Hospital because the latter is relatively far and one whole morning is required to be spent at the hospital, which they can ill-afford.

Secondly, in some government or charitable hospitals nurses and ward boys exploit the helpless patients for providing the latter with bedsheets and other such articles.

Thirdly, ignorance of certain services led to their non-utilization.

(iii) Major Social Problems in India

The participants were less participative here as compared to the earlier two themes. Women mentioned poverty, illiteracy, low status of women and unemployment as the major social problems. Interestingly, they mentioned that poverty is not too grave a problem provided one knows how to spend the available income intelligently. They were also able to see that most problems are related and caused by one another.

Concerning low status of women, it was concluded that women themselves would have to fight for achieving higher status by becoming literate and independent. There is sound social legislation to support them.

Evaluation : Today it was a little serious business contrasted against three previous story telling sessions. The women also appeared unsure how 'major social problems' discussion merited a place in our health education programme. We had included it with a view that some other topical issues also be discussed in addition to the main theme.

Session-XI

Date : 11-9-1987
Time : 2.30 To 4.30 p.m.

Objective : (i) Demonstration of a nutritive snack- 'Poona Bhel'.
(ii) Discussion of modification of some cookery practices for conserving nutritive value of cooked food.
(iii) Guidelines for fuel conservation

Media Used : (i) Cookery demonstration
(ii) Group discussion.

Process and Observations: This idea was borrowed from a programme conducted in one anganwadi by an ICDS worker. In this session too we had a guest volunteer as person in charge of the session. The guest volunteer had brought sprouted whole grain cereals of four kinds and other ingredients which are used in preparation of ordinary 'bhel'. Nutritive value of ordinary 'bhel' is increased manifold by adding sprouted whole grain cereals and curds to it without losing its taste.

The guest volunteer engaged the women in informal conversation to explain to them the recipe under demonstration, scientific methods of daily cooking to conserve nutritive value of foodstuffs, ways to economics fuel consumption and how routine meals can be fortified by simple modifications.

Women actively helped in the preparation and the guest volunteer gave them importance by saying that the former were well experienced in cooking and could evolve new recipes themselves.

At the end of the demonstration all had a helping of the snack.

Evaluation : The latent objective of having a 'lighter session' and some refreshment for the group were well served. How far the women would adopt scientific ways of cooking in their daily lives remains to be seen. But in this session they were equipped with the necessary knowledge.

Session-XII

Date : 7-10-1987
Time : 2.30 To 4.00 p.m.

Objective : (i) To impart knowledge about the term 'immunity' and immunization schedule.
(ii) To inquire from women whether and what reservations they harboured against immunizing their children.

Media Used : (i) Immunization Chart
(ii) Group discussion.

Process and Observation: To begin with purpose of the session and some background knowledge of immunization was given by lecture method. Group discussion method was used to clarify the term immunity, explain immunization schedule and know their reservations against immunization.

An immunization chart in Gujarati language was used for illustration. Most women knew about vaccines but they found it difficult to comprehend the time factor and the disease against which a particular vaccine provides protection.

Regarding their reservations against immunization, some women said that someone known to them had grave side effects or abcess at the site of the injection (perhaps the syringe was not properly sterilised). Few also said that it is 'not done' in their family.

Evaluation : Though the women listened with interest, it was obvious that this one session on the subject would be inadequate. It was decided to organise a film show on 'immunization' for building their knowledge further.

Session-XIII

Date : 8-10-1987
Time : 4.30 To 5.30 p.m.

Objective	: To emphasize upon the importance of immunization in the minds of participants and other community members at an effective level.
Media Used	: A rally by community children carrying relevant posters in a child-to-child approach.

Process and Observations: This session was a surprise item for participant women in our health education programme. We were successful in training some community children to walk together in a rally, carry posters and shout slogans on immunization. It was planned as a logical sequel to the group discussion on immunization on the previous day. The main purpose was to dramatically present importance of immunization to the entire community as this was an extremely important issue.

Field work students were assigned the responsibility of preparing suitable posters which they had procured from the Paediatrics department of S.S.G. Hospital, Vadodara and training the children for the rally. The theme of posters and slogans as translated from vernacular were-

(i) Key to Child Health-
Give the Vaccine
Arrest the Disease
(ii) Immunization is the Birthright of your Children.
(iii) We want Immunization.

Evaluation : The new techniques seemed to have made the intended impact.

Session-XIV

Date : 16-10-1987
Time : 3.00 To 4.30 p.m.

Objective : To organise a film show on the theme of immunization.

Media Used : (i) Film show

(ii) Group discussion.

Materials : (i) Projector and other equipments were secured from Information Department, as also their technician.

(ii) Film was obtained from Baroda Citizens Council, a voluntary organisation in the field of Urban Community Work.

Process and Observations: This was one session in which we had made a massive blunder albeit un-knowingly and despite careful planning. We had intended to screen a film on immunization and contacted B.C.C. for the purpose. We were told that such a film is available but we should make our own arrangements for the equipment.

Having done the latter, one of the field work students collected the film cassette which the B.C.C. worker gave. On the outer jacket of the cassette there was a slip saying that inside there was a film on immunization.

However, when the operator began to project the film it turned out to be one on the oft-repeated theme of family planning. The interventionists were simply shocked and the participants visibly disappointed. Anyway, it was too late to do anything about it then, we continued screening the film out of respect for the personnel from Information Department and our field work students who had taken pains to organise it.

Obviously, we dispensed with the earlier planned follow-up discussion.

Evaluation : We learnt a costly lesson. It showed how an ill-conceived theme is rejected by a clientele group. Indeed, in the episode today the theme was well chosen and good planning was also made. Yet due to circumstances beyond our control, the presentation failed.

Session-XV

Date : 27-2-1987

Time : 3.30 To 5.00 p.m.

Objective : Valedictory function and award of Certificates and Prizes to the participants.

Process and Observations: The participants evinced keen interest in the function from the very beginning. They demanded that some 'important person' must be invited and that they were ready to present a prayer song at the beginning and a 'garba dance' at the end. When we told them that the faculty agency-F.S.K.K. would provide light refreshments they were very happy. Immediately the women suggested that they would themselves prepare some 'nutritious snack' and tea. It was our turn to feel pleased.

Subsequently, Assistant Professor in Pharmacology, Medical College, Vadodara was invited as the chief guest. Other preparations of arranging for a traditional lamp, garlands, decoration of balwadi, writing of certificates and purchase of prizes was done with the help of field work students.

Kanuben and Neeruben undertook the responsibility of prayer song, 'garba' dance and refreshments.

The participants garlanded the chief guest, student workers and the researcher at the beginning and a prayer followed. The chief guest lighted the traditional lamp as a symbolic gesture and later awarded the certificates and prizes as announced by a field work student. A special prize was awarded to Kanuben for her meritorious services. To our immense satisfaction there were no misunderstandings amongst the participants regarding our selection of awardees for various prizes. The chief guest at the end informally chatted with the participants praising them and also inquiring what they had learnt. Next the ladies presented a lively 'garba' dance which everyone enjoyed.

In the very end Neeruben proposed a formal vote of thanks and snacks were served.

Evaluation : The women conducted themselves maturedly and discharged all the responsibilities volunteered for by them in a commendable way. This is worth mentioning because it reflects growth in their personalities as a side gain of the health education programme. The women felt a tremendous sense of achievement which was evident from their active involvement in planning of this session ab initio.

SECTION 5.2

RESULTS BASED ON HYPOTHESIS TESTING

It may be recalled here that in order to study the impact of HEP, the researcher had postulated six hypotheses numbered 8 to 13 as given in section 1.6.3. An assessment of the same, based on Student's t-test and findings of correlation and multiple regression analysis to establish the nature of relationship between knowledge, attitudes and practices of health care of underfives amongst mothers and some relevant predictor variables would be presented serially in this section.

5.2.1 *Hypothesis 8: The mean scores of knowledge in each unit pertaining to health care of underfives amongst treatment group mothers would show increase after the HEP vis-a-vis the corresponding values before*

The knowledge content in the KAP scale contained thirteen component units as per below:

Knowledge of Diarrhoea
" " Measles
" " Chicken Pox
" " Anaemia
" " Tetanus
" " Scabies
" " Infants feeding
" " Nutritious diet
" " Ante-natal care
" " Post-natal care
" " Immunization
" " Family Planning
" " Health Services in the neighbourhood and at city level.

Correspondingly, hypothesis 8 could be treated as a composite of thirteen sub-parts each of which represented one of the above stated units. Before-after paired samples' t-test analysis of these sub-parts have been presented serially in tables and numbered as 5.1, 5.2, 5.3, 5.4, 5.5, 5.6, 5.7 and 5.8.

5.2.1.1 *Knowledge of Common Childhood Diseases*

Table 5.1 presents results pertaining to the knowledge scores with respect to the common childhood diseases covered in HEP. Regarding each disease the women were taught about its usual seasons of occurrence, common symptoms, complications and harmful effects, disease management and disease prevention. The table displays that the mean score increase in case of knowledge of diarrhoea, measles, chicken pox, tetanus, and Scabies were highly significant at p levels of 0 per cent, 0 per cent, 1.3 per cent, .1 per cent and .1 per cent respectively. Only in the case of anaemia the mean increase was not significant as the 2-tail probability

TABLE 5.1: t-test Analysis: Pre and Post-Intervention Mean Scores of Knowledge Regarding Childhood Diseases in Treatment Group

n of cases: 13

Degrees of Freedom: 12

Information	Time of Measurement	Mean	S.D	Correl-ation	t-value	2-Tail Prob
Diarrhoea	Pre	2.6154	1.121	.265	–5.58	
				.265	–5.58	.000* .1
	Post	5.9231	2.139			
Measles	Pre	4.0000	1.472			
				.101	–4.85	.000* .2
	Post	6.8462	1.676			
Chicken Pox	Pre	3.4615	1.613			
				.557	–2.91	.013* .3
	Post	5.1538	2.1538			
Anaemia	Pre	.4615	1.198			
				.657	–1.47	0.168* .4
	Post	1.1538	2.230			
Tetanus	Pre	.6923	.947			
				.043	–4.57	.001*.5
	Post	4.6154	2.987			
Scabies	Pre	.3846	.768			
				.141	–4.38	.001*.6
	Post	2.2308	1.423			

*.1 Extremely Significant at 0%
*.2 " " 0%
*.3 " " 1.3%
*.4 Not " 16.8% – As above 5% is not significant.
*.5 Extremely Significant at .1%
*.6 " " .1%

value was .168.

Story-telling sessions followed by group discussions were the media of instruction used here. The literature with illustrated pictorial presentation was obtained from Sarabhai Science Centre and three volunteers from the learners' group read aloud the stories in three different sessions. One such illustrated story on Diarrhoea has been given in appendix for reference purposes. The sessions were immensely enjoyed by the participants and as the results show, the medium of story-telling was found to be highly effective too, except indeed in case of Anaemia.

5.2.1.2 *Knowledge of Infant Feeding*

TABLE 5.2 : t-test Analysis: Pre and Post-Intervention Mean Scores of Knowledge Regarding Infant Feeding in Treatment Group

Variable Code

V_{24}: Pre-Intervention Mean Score Knowledge of Infant Feeding.

V_{25} : Post-Intervention Mean Score Knowledge of Infant Feeding.

n of Cases : 13

Degrees of Freedom : 12

Variable	Mean	S.D.	Correlation	t-value	2-Tail Prob.
V_{24}	16.0000	5.538			
			.235	– 7.27	.000*
V_{25}	29.6923	5.437			

* Extremely Signification at 0%

Table 5.2 depicts analysis of change in knowledge of infant feeding. The mean scores rose from 16.0000 to 29.6923 under the impact of HEP and the increase was highly significant at p=.000 level. In this area the women were expected to possess fair level of knowledge before intervention and sure enough it was so (in relative terms). Therefore, quiz type games were specially designed to help women learn more about colostrum and why it should be given to the newborn; breast-milk although a complete food in early infanthood needs to be supplemented by solid foods soon later at the correct weaning age; nutritive and cheap weaning foods; special nutritional requirements of infants and importance of maintaining cleanliness while feeding. The technique of games yielded positive results and much could be accomplished in a short time of one session.

5.2.1.3 *Knowledge of Nutritious Diet*

TABLE 5.3 : t-test Analysis: Pre and Post-Intervention Mean Scores of Knowledge Regarding Nutritious Diet in Treatment Group

Variable Code

V_{42} : Pre-Intervention Mean Score Knowledge of Nutritious Diet.

V_{43} : Post-Intervention Mean Score Knowledge of Nutritious Diet.

n of Cases: 13

Degrees of Freedom: 12

Variable	Mean	S.D	Correlation	t-value	2-Tail Prob.
V_{42}	3.4615	1.330			
			.904	–2.13	054*
V_{43}	3.8462	1.519			

* Significant at 5.4%

Table 5.3 presents analysis of change in knowledge of nutritious diet. This unit of information was found to be the most difficult one to comprehend by the learners' group. The particulars covered under this head were-rich sources of vitamins A, B, C and D, Calcium, Iron and Proteins; their broad functions; harmful effects caused by their deficiencies and finally the concept of a balanced meal. A reference was also made to role of fats, carbohydrates and other minerals but it was kept to a brief minimum lest the participants get confused. The communication techniques used were lectures aided by charts and posters, group discussion, notes presentation by a participant and finally a quiz game. Nearly three and half sessions were required. As the statistics reveal mean score of knowledge of nutritious diet rose from 3.4615 to 3.8462 under the impact of the combined efforts at imparting this education. However, the mean increase narrowly missed the level of significance at $p<.05$ as the 2-tail probability value was .054.

5.2.1.4 *Knowledge of Ante-natal Care*

TABLE 5.4 : t-test Analysis: Pre and Post Intervention Mean Scores of Knowledge Regarding Pre-Natal Care in Treatment Group.

Variable Code

V_{30} : Pre-Intervention Mean Score Knowledge of Pre-Natal Care.

V_{31} : Post-Intervention Mean Score Knowledge of Pre-Natal Care.

n of Cases: 13

Degrees of Freedom: 12

Variable	Mean	S.D	Correlation	t-value	2-Tail Prob.
V_{30}	13.0000	3.894			
			.388	–5.17	.000*
V_{31}	19.6154	4.407			

* Extremely Significant at 0%

Table 5.4 depicts impact of HEP knowledge of ante-natal care. The package of information included importance of regular medical examination; correct diet of a pregnant mother, importance of light exercise as well as sleep and relaxation, correct postures, schedule and importance of tetanus toxoid immunization. The communication techniques used was a talk by a lady Gynaecologist from S.S.G. Hospital, Baroda. The pre-intervention mean score rose from 13.0000 to 19.6154 and the difference was highly significant at 0 per cent level since the 2-tail probability value was .000. It needs to be mentioned here that the guest speaker was much impressed by the intellectual curiosity displayed by the participants and their awareness regarding weaning, nutritious food and family planning etc. the topics which the doctor discussed initially to 'warm-up' the session.

5.2.1.5 *Knowledge of Post-natal Care*

TABLE 5.5 : t-test Analysis: Pre and Post-Intervention Mean Scores of Knowledge Regarding Post-Natal Care in Treatment Group

Variable Code

V_{32} : Pre-Intervention Mean Score Knowledge of Post-Natal Care.

V_{33} : Post-Intervention Mean Score Knowledge of Post-Natal Care.

n of Cases: 13

Degrees of Freedom: 12

Variable	Mean	S.D	Correlation	t-value	2-Tail Prob.
V_{32}	.6923	.480			
			.413	– 8.80	.000*
V_{33}	2.4615	.776			

* Extremely Significant at 0%

Table 5.5 reveals analysis of change in knowledge of post-natal care. The information covered here was importance of medical examination of the mother and child after delivery and spacing of future births. The same lady Gynaecologist who gave a talk on ante-natal care spoke on this subject too. In fact both topics were covered by her in a single session.

It can be seen from the table that mean score knowledge of participants rose from .6923 to 2.4615, the difference being highly significant at 0% level as the 2-tail probability value was .000.

5.2.1.6 *Knowledge of Immunization*

TABLE 5.6 : t-test Analysis: Pre and Post-Intervention Mean Scores of Knowledge Regarding Immunization in Treatment Group.

Variable Code

V_{50} : Pre-Intervention Mean Score Knowledge of Immunization

V_{51} : Post-Intervention Mean Score Knowledge of Immunization

n of Cases: 13

Degrees of Freedom: 12

Variable	Mean	S.D	Correlation	t-value	2-Tail Prob.
V_{50}	3.9231	2.532			
			.264	– 5.96	.000*
V_{43}	18.6154	7.547			

* Extremely Significant at 0%

Table 5.6 depicts change in knowledge of immunization. Information imparted under this head included importance of immunization, its schedule and which vaccine provides protection against what illness. Three techniques, namely, lecture aided by charts, group discussion and a childrens' rally at the end of the session in child-to-child approach were used. While the former two methods helped women learn more about immunization at a cognitive level and also clarify some of their misgivings about the same; the rally achieved its intended aim of an appeal to the community as a whole at an affective level of learning about the importance of immunization. About 25 community children were quietly (without the knowledge of elders) trained to carry posters and shout slogans like—

'We want Immunization'
'Immunization Is the Birthright of Children'
'Give the Vaccine-Arrest The Disease'

The overall impact of the teaching methods was spectacular as shown in the table. The mean score rose from 3.9231 to 18.6154. The mean difference was highly significant at p= 0% level since the two-tail probability value was .000.

5.2.1.7 *Knowledge of Family Planning*

TABLE 5.7 : t-test Analysis: Pre and Post-Intervention Mean Scores of Knowledge Regarding Family Planning in Treatment Group

Variable Code

V_{34}: Pre-Intervention Mean Score Knowledge of Family Planning.

V_{43} : Post-Intervention Mean Score Knowledge of Family Planning.

n of Cases: 13

Degrees of Freedom: 12

Variable	Mean	S.D	Correlation	t-value	2-Tail Prob.
V_{34}	14.8462	5.226			
			.549	– 5.78	.000*
V_{35}	24.4615	6.972			

* Extremely Significant at 0%

Table 5.7 depicts change in knowledge of family planning. Two sessions were devoted to communicate about the advantages of limiting family size, proper spacing of births, temporary and permanent methods of contraception, difficulties and side-effects of different methods. Two techniques, namely, story-telling with flip charts and a film show were used. The illustrated story material was obtained from K.G. Childrens' Hospital, Baroda and a student social worker presented it. Film show was arranged with the help of the State Information Department and Baroda Citizens' Council. The film show was not much appreciated by the participants as they expressed that a recreational film would have been more welcome. However, the score knowledge rose from 14.8462 to 24.4615, which was highly significant difference, at 0 per cent level since the 2-tail probability value was .000.

5.2.1.8 *Knowledge of Health Services*

TABLE 5.8 : t-test Analysis: Pre and Post-Intervention Mean Scores of Knowledge Regarding Health Services

Variable Code

V_{48} : Pre-Intervention Mean Score Knowledge of Health Services.

V_{49} : Post-Intervention Mean Score Knowledge of Health Services.

n of Cases: 13

Degrees of Freedom: 12

Variable	Mean	S.D	Correlation	t-value	2-Tail Prob.
V_{48}	2.6154	.650			
			.447	-2.95	.018*
V_{49}	4.3846	1.044			

* Extremely Significant at 1.8%

Table 5.8 depicts the change in knowledge of health services. During one session, a lecture followed by group discussion sought to upgrade women's awareness of immunization, ante-natal, post-natal, family planning and general curative services available both in the neighbourhood and at city level. The Mean scores rose from 2.6154 to 4.3846 and the difference was significant at 1.8 per cent level since the two-tailed probability value was .018.

5.2.1.9 *Status of Hypothesis and After HEP*

As brought out by the on-going discussion, hypothesis 8 was found to be highly acceptable on eleven of its component thirteen sub-items. Of the remaining two, the level of significance for mean change in knowledge of nutritious diet was narrowly missed at $p < .05$ level as the 2-tail probability value was .054. Only in case of change in knowledge of Anaemia the 2-tail probability value of .168 was much away from the acceptable level of significance. In overall terms, therefore, it is justified that hypothesis 8 be accepted and retained.

5.2.2 *Hypothesis 9: The mean Scores of Knowledge in each unit pertaining to health care of underfives amongst treatment group mothers would be higher than scores obtained by the control group after HEP*

As explained earlier in the case of hypothesis 8, hypothesis 9 could be treated as a composite of the same thirteen sub-units as presented in section 5.2.1 (For details please refer section 5.2.1). Results of change in knowledge in all the component units as shown in table No. 5.9 and their presentation now would follow the same pattern as in the previous sections. Also since the contents covered and the communication techniques are the same as in case of H8, the information would not be repeated here.

TABLE 5.9 : t-test Analysis: Pre and Post-Intervention Mean Scores of Knowledge Regarding Health Care of Underfives in Treatment and Control Groups.

Information	Time of Measurement	Group	Mean	S.D	F Value	t Value	Degrees of Freedom	2-Tail Prob.
Diarrhoea	Pre	Trt. n=13	2.6154	1.121				
					1.68	.35	26	.728
		Cont. n=15	3.567	1.033				
	Post	Trt. n=13	5.9231	2.139				
					3.15	1.49	17.93	.048
		Cont. n=15	4.0614	1.163				
Measles	Pre	Trt. n=13	4.0000	1.472				
					1.10	-1.10	26	.280
		Cont. n=15	4.6000	1.404				
	Post	Trt. n=13	6.8462	1.676				
					1.17	2.37	26	.140
		Cont. n=15	5.4000	1.549				

Information	Time of Measure-ment	Group	Mean	S.D	F Value	t Value	Degrees of Freedom	2-Tail Prob.
Chicken Pox	Pre	Trt. n=13	3.4615	1.613				
					1.15	–.11	26	.911
		Cont. n=15	3.5333	1.727				
	Post	Trt. n=13	5.1538	2.512				
					1.64	1.52	26	.140
		Cont. n=15	3.8667	1.959				
Anaemia	Pre	Trt. n=15	.4615	1.198				
					Computer Warning: No Variance for Independent Samples t-test			
		Cont. n=15	.0000	.000				
	Post	Trt. n=13	1.1538	2.230				
					74.62	1.75	12.28	.106
		Cont. n=15	.0667	.258				
Tetanus	Pre	Trt. n=13	.6923	.947				
					3.42	–1.10	22.11	.284
		Cont. n=15	1.2667	1.751				
	Post	Trt. n=13	4.6154	1.987				
					3.05	3.57	18.50	.002
		Cont. n=15	1.2667	1.710				
Scabies	Pre	Trt. n=13	.3846	.768				
					3.88	–1.38	21.37	.181
		Cont. n=15	1.0000	1.512				
	Post	Trt. n=13	2.2308	1.423				
					1.61	1.34	26	.193
		Cont. n=15	1.4000	1.805				

Information	Time of Measurement	Group	Mean	S.D	F Value	t Value	Degrees of Freedom	2-Tail Prob.
Infant feeding	Pre	Trt. n=13	16.0000	5.538	1.31	2.24	26	.034
		Cont. n=15	11.6000	4.837				
	Post	Trt. n=13	29.6923	5.437	1.32	7.33	26	.000
		Cont. n=15	15.6000	4.733				
Nutritious Diet	Pre	Trt. n=13	3.4615	1.330	1.41	-.30	26	.767
		Cont. n=15	3.6000	1.121				
	Post	Trt. n=13	3.8462	1.519	1.67	.35	26	.728
		Cont. n=15	3.6667	1.175				
Ante-natal Care	Pre	Trt. n=13	9.6154	4.407	1.98	1.84	26	.123
		Cont. n=15	8.2667	4.992				
	Post	Trt. n=13	13.0000	3.894	1.08	3.98	26	.000
		Cont. n=15	9.0672	4.053				
Post-natal	Pre	Trt. n=13	.6923	.480	1.10	-.23	26	.819
		Cont. n=15	.7333	.480				
	Post	Trt. n=13	2.4615	.776	2.88	7.04	18.85	.000
		Cont. n=15	.7333	.458				

Information	Time of Measurement	Group	Mean	S.D	F Value	t Value	Degrees of Freedom	2-Tail Prob.
Immunization	Pre	Trt. n=13	3.9231	2.532				
					1.06	.60	26	.551
		Cont. n=15	3.3333	2.610				
	Post	Trt. n=13	18.6154	7.547				
					2.21	5.62	20.55	.000
		Cont. n=15	4.7333	5.077				
Family Planning	Pre	Trt. n=13	8.8974	5.226				
					1.94	1.81	26	.120
		Cont. n=15	7.6000	6.685				
	Post	Trt. n=13	24.4615	6.972				
					1.16	5.64	26	.000
		Cont. n=15	8.9333	7.507				
Health Services	Pre	Trt. n=13	2.6154	.650				
					1.03	.34	26	.740
		Cont. n=15	2.5333	1.040				
	Post	Trt. n=13	4.3846	1.044				
					2.01	5.15	21.21	.000
		Cont. n=15	2.6000	.737				

5.2.2.1 *Knowledge of Common Childhood Diseases*

Information of Six Childhood diseases, namely, diarrhoea, measles, chicken pox, anaemia, tetanus and scabies in Table 5.9. appears under two sub-heads with respect to the time of measurement. It can be seen from Table 5.9 that the pre-intervention mean scores in treatment and control group with regard to all the six diseases when subjected to independent samples t-test were found to be not at all significant at $p<.05$ level since the 2-tail probability values were much higher. In other words, the two groups before intervention were well matched and highly comparable as required. (In fact, in case of anaemia, the pre-intervention means had hardly and variance as per the computer warning) However, post intervention t-test results show that in case of diarrhoea, measles and tetanus the information gained by treatment group under impact of HEP was highly significant at 4.8 per cent, 2.5 per cent, .2 per cent and 0 per cent respectively. The mean difference (post intervention) was not significant enough in case of chicken pox, anaemia and scabies as the two-tail probability values were high.

5.2.2.2 *Knowledge of Infant Feeding*

Information on infant feeding in Table 5.9 appears under two sub-heads with respect to the time of measurement. Pre intervention data shows that mean scores in the treatment and control groups were significantly different at 3.4 per cent level. Therefore, this was the odd case in which the two groups were not well matched and comparable as required by an experimental study. However, the post intervention data reveals that although the means of both the groups increased during the intervention, perhaps due to 'the trickle around' effect, the mean of treatment group rose spectacularly and the t-test result this time was highly significant as the 2-tail probability value was .000. To that extent, it can be said with confidence that our HEP produced positive change in knowledge of infant feeding.

5.2.2.3 *Knowledge of Nutritious Diet*

Information on knowledge of nutritious diet in Table 5.9 clearly depicts that the two groups were initially well matched and highly comparable as required. However, the knowledge gain by treatment group under HEP was not significantly different from control group mothers as the 2-tail probability value under independent samples was .728 well beyond the $p<.05$ level of significance. Earlier, in case of hypothesis 8, the results of the before-after t-test had brought out a significant change in knowledge in treatment group itself. The failure of t-test under hypothesis 9, is perhaps a pointer 'to trickle around' effect of knowledge passed on by treatment group mothers towards their friends in the control group. It is not at all a surprising matter in a small and compact geographical area.

5.2.2.4 *Knowledge of Ante-natal Care*

Information of ante-natal care as shown in Table 5.9 conforms to the research expectation that the treatment and control groups be well matched and comparable before intervention since pre-intervention 2 tail probability value was .123. At the post-intervention stage the mean scores of the two groups were significantly different, since the 2-tail probability value was .000. To that extent, hypothesis 9 is acceptable.

5.2.2.5 *Knowledge of Post-natal Care*

Table 5.9 clearly depicts that the pre intervention mean scores in treatment and control groups with respect to knowledge of post-natal care were highly comparable and the two groups were well matched as the 2-tail probability value under independent samples t-test was .123 which is not significant at $p<.05$ level. Hence, the required condition for experimental research was satisfactorily met with. t-test analysis of post intervention mean scores was found to be highly significant at 0 per cent level since the two-tail probability value was .000. Hence, the HEP was impactful in this respect too.

5.2.2.6 *Knowledge of Immunization*

Table 5.9 reveals that t-test analysis of mean scores of knowledge of immunization in treatment and control groups was not significant at $p<.05$ level since the 2 tail probability value was .551. In other words, the groups were well matched and highly comparable as required. The post intervention independent samples t-test was found to be highly significant at 0 per cent level since the 2-tail probability value was .000. To that extent, the hypothesis is acceptable.

5.2.2.7 *Knowledge of Family Planning*

Pre-intervention data on family planning as shown in Table 5.9 depicts that the treatment and control groups were well matched and highly comparable at that time as required since the 2-tail probability value was .120, well beyond the desired level of significance. However, the post-intervention data conforms to the hypothesis 9 since the 2-tail probability value here was .000 the level of significance being extremely high at 0 per cent. Hence, the HEP was impactful in this unit, too.

5.2.2.8 *Knowledge of Health Services*

Information of health services in Table 5.9 reveals that the pre intervention and post-intervention mean scores in treatment and control groups conform to hypothesis 9. The two groups were highly well matched before intervention as the 2-tail probability value was .740 well beyond $p<.05$ level of significance. On the other hand, the post-intervention 2-tail probability value was highly significant at 0 per cent. The HEP induced the desired positive changes in this unit as well.

5.2.2.9 *Status of Hypothesis 9 after HEP*

The ongoing presentation in section 5.2.2.1 to 5.2.2.8 brings out that the knowledge gain by participants of HEP was well beyond $p<.05$ level of significance with respect to nine out of thirteen component units. The four units in which the hypothesis stands rejected were knowledge of chicken pox, anaemia, scabies, and nutritious diet. How do we account for this?

The foremost logical deduction would be that our teaching efforts were inadequate and inefficient. Perhaps more concentrated inputs were required. But when we compare these results with the results of hypothesis 8 which also represented the very same thirteen knowledge units for which the teaching contents and techniques were also the same, we find that hypothesis 8 was untenable only in case of knowledge of anaemia and in fact it narrowly missed 5 per cent level of significance by .4 per cent. This implies that in the present case if the t-test results are found to be non-significant it was more because of simultaneous knowledge gain by the control group members rather than due to insufficient knowledge gain by treatment group. This is most likely to have happened because the two groups did not exist in isolation. In fact they were both drawn from the same compact geographical area. The treatment group women had probably shared their learnings from the HEP sessions with their neighbours and friends from control group and knowledge trickled across. Although it upset hypothesis 9, spread of correct knowledge is certainly a desirable trend.

Taking all aspects into consideration, therefore, it seems reasonable to retain hypothesis 9, making allowances for side effects of working in an open community setting.

5.2.3 *Hypothesis 10: The mean scores of attitudes (in each unit) pertaining to health care of underfives amongst treatment group mothers would show increase after the HEP vis-a-vis the corresponding values before*

The attitude content in the KAP scale contained three component units as per below:

Attitude to Infant feeding
Attitude to Women and Female child
Attitude to Health Professionals

Correspondingly, hypothesis 10, could be treated as a composite of three sub-units, each of which represents one of the above stated content. Before-after paired samples t-test tables numbered as 5.10, 5.11, 5.12.

5.2.3.1 *Attitude to Infant Feeding*

TABLE 5.10 : t-test Analysis: Pre and Post Intervention Mean Scores of Attitudes Towards Infant Feeding in Treatment Group

Variable Code

V_{26} - Pre-Intervention Mean Score Attitudes Towards Infant Feeding.

V_{27} - Post-Intervention Mean Score Attitude Towards Infant Feeding.

n of Cases: 13

Degrees of Freedom: 12

Variable	Mean	S.D	Correlation	t value	2-Tail Prob.
V_{26}	2.4615	1.198			
			.221	– 2.28	042*
V_{27}	3.4619	1.330			

* Significant at 4.2%

In this sub-section, our strategy was to help women develop positive attitudes by first correcting their false beliefs or add to their knowledge on issues like whether colostrum should be given to the new-born infant or discarded; whether an infant should be fed as and when he/she cries or periodically as per schedule; whether timely weaning is necessary for child health or not and whether feeding water is important.

It can be seen from table 5.10 that the mean scores of attitudes in the treatment group rose from 2.4615 to 3.4619 and the change was significant at 4.2 per cent level.

Hence hypothesis 10 is acceptable in this case.

5.2.3.2 *Attitude to Women and Female Child*

TABLE 5.11 : t-test Analysis: Pre and Post Intervention Mean Score Attitudes Towards Women and Female Children in Treatment Groups

Variable Code:

V_{44} - Pre-Intervention Mean Score Attitudes Towards Women and Female Child.

V_{45} - Post-Intervention Mean Score Attitudes Towards Women and Female child.

n of Cases: 13

Degrees of Freedom: 12

Variable	Mean	S.D	Correlation	t value	2-Tail Prob.
V_{44}	1.0769	.641			
			.186	–3.86	.008*
V_{45}	2.8462	.689			

* Extremely Significant at .8%

In this sub-section, issues like whether daughters are a burden; whether two sons in each family are preferable; whether there should be at least one son in each family; why life expectancy amongst women is lower that men; why greater number of male patients seek medical care as compared to female patients were dealt with. Before-after analysis of mean scores of attitudes as shown in Table 5.11 reflects that the change was highly significant at .8 per cent level since the 2-tail probability value was .008.

Hence, the hypothesis is tenable with respect to attitudes towards women and female child.

5.2.3.3 *Attitudes to Health Professionals*

TABLE 5.12 : t-test Analysis: Pre and Post-Intervention Mean Scores of Attitudes Towards Health Professionals in Treatment Group

Variable Code:

V_{46} - Pre-Intervention Mean Score Attitudes Towards Health Professionals.

V_{47} - Post-Intervention Mean Score Attitudes Towards Health Professionals.

n of Cases: 13

Degrees of Freedom: 12

Variable	Mean	S.D	t value	2-Tail	Prob.
V_{46}	2.3077	1.377			
			.488	-2.65	.025*
V_{47}	3.3846	.768			

* Significant at 2.5%

In this sub-section, attitudes of women towards health professionals like doctors, nurses, vaccinators, family planning workers and social workers were probed into both before and after intervention. Table 5.12 illustrates that the mean score rise with respect to attitudes to health professionals was significant at 2.5 per cent level of significance since the 2-tail probability value was .025.

Hence the hypothesis is tenable in this case, too.

5.2.3.4 *Status of Hypothesis 10 after HEP*

The on-going presentation in section 5.2.3.1, 5.2.3.2 and 5.2.3.3 brings out that the hypothesis 10 was tenable with respect to all the three component units of the attitudes content in the KAP scale.

Hence, hypothesis 10 is found to be un-ambiguously acceptable and stands retained.

5.2.4 *Hypothesis 11: The mean scores of attitudes (in each unit) pertaining to health care of underfives amongst treatment group mothers would be higher than control group mothers' scores after the HEP*

As explained earlier in the case of hypothesis 10, hypothesis 11 can also be treated as a composite of the same three sub-units as presented in section 5.2.3 (For details please refer section 5.2.3). Results of change in attitudes in all the component units as shown in Table 5.13 and their presentation here would follow the same pattern as in the previous sections. Also since the contents covered are the same as in the case of hypothesis 10, the information would not be repeated here.

5.2.4.1 *Attitude to Infant Feeding*

Information on infant feeding in Table 5.13 reveals that the treatment and control groups were well matched and highly comparable before intervention as the 2-tail probability value was .648. In other words, the required research condition that the two groups be near equals before intervention was satisfactorily met with. However, the post intervention t-test analysis of the mean scores of the two groups show that the treatment group mothers had undergone an attitudinal change which was significant at 4.7 per cent level since the 2-tail probability value was .047. Hence, the HEP was impactful in this case.

5.2.4.2 *Attitude to Women and Female Child*

Table 5.13 depicts that pre intervention mean scores in treatment and control groups with respect to attitudes towards women and female child were highly comparable and the two groups were well matched as the 2-tail probability value under independent samples t-test was .968. Hence, the required condition for experimental research was satisfactorily met with. The t-test analysis of post intervention mean scores was found to be highly significant at 0 per cent level since the 2-tail probability value was .000. Hence, the HEP was impactful in this respect too.

TABLE 5.13 : t-test Analysis: Pre and Post-Intervention Mean Scores of Attitudes Towards Health Care of Underfives Amongst Treatment and Control Groups

Information	Time of Measurement	Group	Mean	S.D	F Value	t Value	Degrees of Freedom	2-Tail Prob.
Infant Feeding	Pre	Trt. n=13	2.4615	1.198				
					1.35	.46	26	.648
		Cont. n=15	2.2667	1.033				
	Post	Trt. n=13	3.5678	1.330				
					1.04	2.04	26	.047
		Cont. n=15	2.5333	1.302				
Women and Female Child	Pre	Trt. n=13	1.0769	.641				
					1.21	.04	26	.968
		Cont. n=15	1.0667	.704				
	Post	Trt. n=13	2.8462	.689				
					1.04	6.74	26	.000
		Cont. n=15	1.0667	.704				
Health Professionals	Pre	Trt. n=13	2.3077	1.377				
					1.36	-.19	26	.850
		Cont. n=15	2.4000	1.183				
	Post	Trt. n=13	3.3846	.768				
					2.34	2.84	24.31	.009
		Cont. n=15	2.3333	1.175				

5.2.4.3 *Attitudes to Health Professionals*

Information on health professionals in Table 5.13 reveals that the pre intervention and post intervention t-test analysis of mean scores in treatment group conform to the experimental research requirement that the two groups should have insignificant variance before and significant variance after intervention was satisfactorily met with. The 2-tail probability value before was .850 and found to be not significant at 5 per cent level while the subsequent value was .009 which was significant at 0.9 per cent level. Hence, the hypothesis 11 was found to be tenable in this case.

5.2.4.4 *Status of Hypothesis 11 after HEP*

The presentation in sections 5.3.4.1, 5.3.4.2 and 5.3.4.3 brings out that the hypothesis 11 was tenable with respect to all the component units of attitudes content in the KAP scale.

Hence, hypothesis 11 is found to be un-ambiguously acceptable and retained.

5.2.5 *Hypothesis 12: The mean scores of practice (in each unit) pertaining to health care of underfives amongst treatment group mothers would show increase after the HEP vis-a-vis the corresponding values before.*

The practice content in the KAP scale contained three component units as per below:

Practice of Care and Management of sick child
Practice of Infant feeding
Practice of Personal Hygiene.

Correspondingly, hypothesis 12 could be treated as a composite of three sub units each of which represents one of the above stated contents. Before-after paired samples' t-test analysis of these units have been presented serially in tables numbered 5.14, 5.15 and 5.16 respectively.

5.2.5.1 *Practice of Care and Management of Sick Child*

TABLE 5.14: t-test Analysis: Pre and Post Intervention Mean Scores of Practice Regarding Care and Management of Sick Child in Treatment Group.

Variable Code:

V_{22} — Pre-Intervention Mean Score Practice of Care and Management of Sick Child.

V_{23} — Post-Intervention Mean Score Practice of Care and Management of Sick Child.

n of Cases: 13

Degrees of Freedom: 12

Variable	Mean	S.D	Correlation	t Value	2-Tail Prob.
V_{22}	8.5385	2.259	.594	-2.88	.014*
V_{23}	10.1538	2.230			

* Extremely Significant at 1.4%

In this section, we dealt with practice like giving fluids to a sick child, ORS mix in case of diarrhoea; cleanliness and hygiene of the patient; giving medicines as per physician's instruction even if the sick child protests, completing the full course of treatment even if symptoms subside and isolating the child in case of such requirement. Pre intervention scores were explored and after imparting information of correct practices through group discussion method, post intervention scores were recorded. It was found that mean score difference in treatment group was significant at 1.4% level since the 2-tail probability as determined by t-test analysis was .014 as shown in table. Hence, the hypothesis was tenable in this instance.

5.2.5.2 *Practice of Infant Feeding*

TABLE 5.15: t-test Analysis: Pre and Post-Intervention Mean Scores of Practice of Infant Feeding in Treatment Group

Variable Code:

V_{28} — Pre-Intervention Mean Score Practice of Infant Feeding

V_{29} — Post-Intervention Mean Score Practice of Infant Feeding.

n of Cases: 13

Degrees of Freedom: 12

Variable	Mean	S.D	Correlation	t Value	2-Tail Prob.
V_{28}	4.4615	1.941	.946	– 1.76	.104*
V_{29}	4.7692	1.787			

* Not Significant above 5% level

In this section, we focussed on the actual change in practice in terms of giving recommended solid foods to infants; following a schedule for feeding and not giving in to demand of the infant or convenience of the mother and feeding of water. Before-after t-test analysis of mean scores of practice in treatment group revealed that the difference was not significant at 5 per cent level of significance since the 2-tail probability was .104. In other words, the HEP was not impactful in this instance.

5.2.5.3 *Practice of personal Hygiene*

TABLE 5.16: t-test Analysis: Pre and Post-Intervention Mean Scores of Practice of Personal Hygiene in Treatment Group

Variable Code:

V_{40} — Pre-Intervention Mean Score Practice of Personal Hygiene.

V_{41} — Post-Intervention Mean Score Practice of Personal Hygiene.

n of Cases: 13

Degrees of Freedom: 12

Variable	Mean	S.D	Correlation	t Value	2-Tail Prob.
V_{40}	10.3846	1.981			
			.562	– 4.13	.001*
V_{41}	12.6923	2.287			

* Extremely Significant at 0.1%

In this section, we focussed on oral and dental hygiene; cleanliness of hair, nails and clothes; regular bathing; washing of hands before taking food and also washing of hands before cooking. Since nothing of the aforesaid personal hygiene items were new and it was expected that all women knew about it at cognitive level, it was decided to approach them at an affective level by organising a stylised skit by community children, again in a child-to-child approach. The text of the skit is given in section 5.1. The strategy used yielded highly significant results as shown in table 5.16 that the 2-tail probability under paired samples t-test was .001. Hence, the HEP was highly impactful in this instance, as well.

5.2.5.4 *Status Hypothesis 12 after HEP*

The presentation in section 5.2.5.1, 5.2.5.2 and 5.2.5.3 brings out that the hypothesis 12 tenable with respect to two out of three component units of practice content in the KAP scale.

Hence, it would be judicious to retain hypothesis 12 partially.

5.2.6 *Hypothesis 13: The mean scores of practice (in each unit) pertaining to health care of underfives amongst treatment group mothers would be higher than the scores obtained by control group mothers after the HEP*

As explained earlier in the case of hypothesis 12, hypothesis 13 can also be treated as a composite of the same three sub-units as presented in section 5.2.5 (For details please refer section 5.2.4). Results of change in practice in all the component units as shown in Table 5.17 and their presentation her would follow the same pattern as in the previous sections. Also since the contents covered and the communication techniques used remain the same, the information would not be repeated here.

TABLE 5.17: t-test Analysis: Pre and Post-Intervention Mean Scores of Practice Regarding Health Care of Underfives in Treatment and Control Groups.

Information	Time of Measurment	Group	Mean	S.D	F Value	t Value	Degrees of Freedom	2-Tail Prob.
Care and Management of Sick Child	Pre	Trt. n=13	8.5385	2.259	3.69	1.73	17.47	.101
		Cont. n=15	7.3333	1.175				
	Post	Trt. n=13	10.1538	2.230	1.59	3.47	26	.002
		Cont. n=15	7.5333	1.767				
Infant Feeding	Pre	Trt. n=13	4.4615	1.941	3.04	1.30	18.52	.209
		Cont. n=15	3.6667	1.113				
	Post	Trt. n=13	4.7692	1.787	2.26	1.55	20.38	.137
		Cont. n=15	3.8667	1.187				
Personal Hygiene	Pre	Trt. n=13	10.3846	1.981	2.42	-1.39	24.13	.176
		Cont. n=15	11.7333	3.081				
	Post	Trt. n=13	12.6923	2.287	2.34	.34	25.05	.735
		Cont. n=15	12.3333	3.244				

5.2.6.1 *Practice of Care and Management of Sick Child*

Table 5.17 clearly depicts that the pre intervention mean scores in treatment and control groups with respect to practice of care and management of the sick child were highly comparable and the two groups were well matched as the 2-tail probability value under independent samples t-test analysis was .101 which is not significant at 5 per cent level. Hence, the required condition for experimental research was satisfactorily met with. However, t-test analysis of post intervention mean scores was found to be highly significant at .2 per cent level since the 2-tail probability value was .002. The HEP was, therefore, impactful in this respect.

5.2.6.2 *Practice of Infant Feeding*

Table 5.17 depicts that the pre intervention mean scores in treatment and control groups with respect to practice of infant feeding were highly comparable and well matched, as the 2-tail probability value under independent samples t-test was .209 which is not significant at 5% level. Hence, the required condition for experimental research was satisfactorily met with. Despite HEP, however, t-test analysis of post intervention mean scores was also found to be not significant at 5 per cent level since the probability value was .137. It may be recalled here that practice of infant feeding had not improved significantly in the treatment group itself since hypothesis 12 was clearly rejected in this regard. The post intervention result in case of hypothesis 13 therefore, is not surprising at all.

Therefore, hypothesis 13 clearly stands rejected in this case.

5.2.6.3 *Practice of Personal Hygiene*

Table 5.17 clearly depicts that the pre intervention mean scores in treatment and control groups with respect to practice of personal hygiene were highly comparable and the two groups were well matched as the 2-tail probability value under independent samples t-test was .176 which is not significant at 5 per cent level. Hence, the required condition for experimental research was satisfactorily met with. Despite HEP however, t-test analysis of post intervention mean scores was found to be not significant at 5 per cent level since the 2-tail probability value was .735.

It may be recalled here that in case of hypothesis 12, the post intervention means of treatment and control group were found to be statistically highly different from each other. Then how do we explain the present result. It can be seen from Table 5.17 that the post intervention mean score in both the groups rose although there were no inputs in the control group. Once again, we attribute this trend to 'trickle around' effect wherein the treatment group mothers shared their learning from the HEP with their neighbours and friends in the community belonging to the control group.

The hypothesis 13 is rejected in this instance without any reservations.

5.2.6.4 *Status of Hypothesis 13 after HEP*

The presentation in section 5.2.6.1, 5.2.6.2 and 5.2.6.3 bring out that hypothesis 13 was found to be untenable with respect to two out of three component units of practice content in the KAP scale.

Hence, hypothesis 13 stands clearly rejected

5.2.7 *Results Based on Correlation and Multiple Regression Analysis*

In addition to measuring the impact of the HEP, we wère interested in studying the nature of relationship between the dependent variables of aggregate scores of knowledge, Attitude and Practice and some relevant independent variables like household size, mother's age, mother's education and per capita monthly income. Multiple Regression Analysis was carried out to serve the stated purpose and the discussion of the results obtained follows.

Correlation and Multiple Regression between Criterion Variable V_{72} *i.e.*, Aggregate Knowledge Score and Predictor Variables as listed below:

Household Size, Mother's Age, Mother's Education and Per Capita Monthly Income.

5.2.7.1 *Correlation and Multiple Regression between Criterion Variable V_{72} i.e Aggregate Knowledge Score and Predictor Variables as listed below:*

TABLE 5.18 : Correlation and Multiple Regression between Criterion Variable V_{72} *i.e.* Aggreegate Knowledge Score and Predictor Variables as listed below :

Variable	Label	Mean	Standard Deviation
V_4	Mother's Age	26.000	3.517
V_5	Mother's Edu. *	1.821	1.090
V_8	Household Size	5.179	1.249

V_9	Per Capita Monthly Income	113.821	54.619

N of cases: 28

Correlation:

	V_4	V_5	V_8	V_9	V_{72}
V_4	1.000	-.135	.506	.406	.064
V_5	-.135	1.000	.079	.223	.536
V_8	.506	.079	1.000	-.197	.110
V_9	.046	.223	-.197	1.000	.148
V_{72}	.064	.536	.110	.148	1.000

Multiple Regression:

Method: Step-wise EQ 1: V_{72} (Aggregate Knowledge Score)

Variables in Equation

Variable	B	SE B	T	Sig T.
V_5	10.25918	3.16889	3.237	.0033
(Constant)	925.99221	6.69550	138.301	-.0000

Variables Not in Equation

Variable	Beta In	Min Toler	T	Sig T.
V_4	.13908	.98172	.827	.4159
V_8	.06853	.99381	.406	.6882
V_9	.02972	.95041	.172	.8650

Multiple R .53601

R Square .28730 or 28.73%

Adjusted R Square .25989

Standard Error 17.95594

Variable Code

1 = Illiterate

2 = One to 5 years of formal education

3 = 6 to 9 years of formal education

4 = 10 to 12 years of formal education

As shown in Table 5.18 all the predictor variables bore a positive correlation with aggregate knowledge score. However, only in the case of mother's education the correlation matrix value was high *i.e.* .536 and therefore, step-wise method was employed for regression analysis. It was confirmed that mother's education made a statistically significant and positive impact on knowledge of participants. In other words, higher the educational level of the mother, greater would be the knowledge gained by her. Since the value of R square, was .28730, variance produced by mother's education level was 28.73 per cent which was quite good.

5.2.7.2 *Correlation and Multiple Regression between Criterion Variable V_{73} i.e. Aggregate Attitude Score and Predictor Variables as listed below:*

Household Size, Mother's Age, Mother's Education and Per Capita Monthly Income.

TABLE 5.19 : Correlation and Multiple Regression Analysis between Criterion Variable V_{73} i.e. Aggregate Attitude Score and Predictor Variables as listed below:

Variable	Label	Mean	Standard Deviation
V_4	Mother's Age	26.000	3.517
V_5	Mother's Edu. *	1.821	1.090
V_8	Household Size	5.179	1.249
V_9	Per Capita Monthly Income	113.821	54.619

Correlation:

	V_4	V_5	V_8	V_9	V_{73}
V_4	1.000	–.135	.506	.046	.031
V_5	–.135	1.000	.079	.223	.224
V_8	.506	.079	1.000	–.197	.073
V_9	.046	.223	–.197	1.000	.085
V_{73}	–.031	.224	.073	.085	1.000

Multiple Regression:

Method: Enter EQ 1: V_{73} i.e. Aggregate Attitude Score.

Variables In Equation

Variable	B	SE B	T	Sig T.
V_9	3.918110E-03	.01486	.264	.7944
V_4	–.05460	.25992	–.210	.8355
V_5	.74278	.73680	1.008	.3239
V_8	.27845	.74361	.374	.7115
(Constant)	1.14306	6.02294	.190	.8511

Multiple R	.25775
R Square	.06644 or 6.64%
Adjusted R Square	–.09592
Standard Error	3.90124

Variable Code

* 1 = Illiterate

2 = One to 5 years of formal education

3 = 6 to 9 years of formal education

4 = 10 to 12 years of formal education

Table 5.19 reveals that only mother's age was negatively correlated with attitude score implying that younger the mother-more positive her attitude towards health concerns of her underfives. Since the matrix value was rather low *i.e.*, -.031, the above stated trend was not confirmed under multiple regression analysis. All the other independent variables bore a positive relationship with attitude score but none exerted any statistically significant influence. Since the study sample was rather small, probably some of the subtle changes could not be gauged in the present intervention model.

5.2.7.2 *Correlation and Multiple Regression between Criterion Variable V_{74} i.e. Aggregate Practice Score and Predictor Variables as listed below:*

Household Size, Mother's Age, Mother's Education and Per Capita Monthly Income.

TABLE 5.20: Correlation and Multiple Regression Analysis between Criterion Variable V_{74} *i.e.* Aggregate Practice Score and Predictor Variables as listed below:

Variable	Label	Mean	Standard Deviation
V_4	Mother's Age	26.000	3.517
V_5	Mother's Edu. *	1.821	1.090
V_8	Household Size	5.179	1.249
V_9	Per Capita Monthly Income	113.821	54.619
	N of cases = 28		

	V_4	V_5	V_8	V_9	V_{74}
V_4	1.000	–.135	.506	.046	-.208
V_5	–.135	1.000	.079	.223	.545
V_8	.506	.079	1.000	–.197	–.360
V_9	.046	.223	–.197	1.000	.441
V_{74}	–.208	.545	.360	.441	1.000

Multiple Regression:

Method: Enter EQ 1: V_{74} i.e. Aggregate Practice Score.

Variables in Equation

Variable	B	SE B	T	Sig T.
V_9	.01409	8.80791E-03	1.599	.1234
V_4	.03502	.15402	.227	.8222
V_5	1.48288	.43659	3.396	.0025
V_8	–.92122	.44063	– 2.091	.0478

(Constant)	2.05598	3.56891	.576	.5702
Multiple R	.72232			
R Square	.52175 or	52.17%		
Adjusted R Square	.43858			
Standard Error	2.31169			

Variable Code

*1 = Illiterate

2 = One to 5 years of formal education

3 = 6 to 9 years of formal education

4 = 10 to 12 years of formal education

Table 5.20 reveals that all the four predictor variables had either positive or negative, although low or medium level correlation with aggregate practice score. More-specifically, correlation matrix values for mother's age, mother's education, household size and per capita monthly income were respectively – .208, .545, – .360 and .441. In other words, younger mothers, better educated ones, smaller households and higher per capita incomes contributed more significantly (than others) towards improvement in practice of health care of underfives children. Multiple Regression analysis further brought out that the relationships of mother's education and household size with aggregate practice score (as stated above) was statistically significant too.

Value of R square was considerably high *i.e.*, 52.17 per cent. Therefore, it can be categorically stated that higher educational level of mother and smaller households are strong predictors of practice of health care of underfives.

6

MAJOR FINDINGS, CONCLUSIONS AND THE EMERGENT MODULE

Selecting a research topic can be an intensely personal and passionate choice especially when one works in an applied area with concrete implications for people's lives-Susskind and Klein (1985: 10). The same two authors further state that for many individuals this choice may involve an attempt to use the discipline of science to examine, modify, validate or promulgate their values and to see whether this scientific process clarifies or enhances what they know 'on a gut level' moving that knowledge from the status of belief in the direction of becoming a fact. These statements beautifully sum up the motivational drive that led the researcher to opt for an experimental study; the choice of ultimate goals (pursued); and the broad course of action followed. How far did we traverse the right path and what lessons were learnt on the way are the two relevant questions that must be answered at the end. In this last chapter, therefore, we begin with a summary of the major findings; followed by some logical conclusions; and finally present our experience based know-how of the module of social intervention adopted.

6.1 Statistical Findings

It may be recalled here that for sake of organised presentation, the entire volume of relevant data used has been presented under three different categories *viz.* The Base-Line Survey, Health and Growth-monitoring Interventions and Health Education Intervention in Chapters 3, 4 and 5 respectively. The same pattern would be followed to summerise presentation of major statistically findings.

6.1.1 *The Base-Line Survey Findings*

The base-line survey of 115 families from Harijanwas and Sardargram pockets of Pensionpura slums in Vadodara, where the field experiment was conducted, addressed itself to the task of determining the demographic and socio-economic conditions of the respondent families and also sought information pertaining to certain factors closely related to health of under-fives *i.e.*, daily diet patterns; actual per day consumption of essential food items; incidence of pregnancy wastage and child mortality; utilization of ante-natal, natal, post-natal and family planning services; age at weaning and types of weaning foods given; and motor and mental developmental testing of children between 0-30 months of age. The results are as follows:

6.1.1.1 *Religion:* A vast majority of families were Hindus *i.e.*, 92.17 per cent followed by Christians-5.22 per cent, Muslims 2.61 per cent.

6.1.1.2 *Caste:* Harijans had the maximum numerical strength *i.e.*, 44.35 per cent and were followed closely by schedule caste/tribes other than Harijans-41.03 per cent. Upper Castes-6.80 per cent and noncastes-7.82 per cent made up the total.

6.1.1.3 *Mother-tongue:* Gujarati led the distribution of families on the basis of mother-tongue-73.91 per cent; the rest being Marathi-13.05 per cent; Hindi-5.22 per cent and 'Any other'-7.82 per cent. 'Any other' category included Punjabi, Sindhi, Tamil and Nepali.

6.1.1.4 *Native Place:* Study revealed that 56.41 per cent belonged to Baroda district. 15.82 per cent families hailed from within Gujarat but districts other than Baroda, and 27.77 per cent had migrated from states other than Gujarat.

6.1.1.5 *Family Type:* Under the study there were 63.07 per cent nuclear families and the rest 36.93 per cent were joint families.

6.1.1.6 *Family Size:* Mean Family Size under the study was found to be 4.91 members with a standard deviation of 1.43 members. Besides, 15.65 per cent families had 2 or 3 members: 55.66 per cent had 4 or 5 members; 23.4 per cent had 6 or 7 members and 5.22 per cent families had 8 or 9 members.

6.1.1.7 *Food consumption Units Per Household:* The mean food consumption units per household was found to be 4.03 with a standard deviation of 1.18. Distribution of households based on this criteria was as follows: 26.08 per cent had 2.0-3.0 units; 28.69 per cent had 3.1-4.0 units; 27.82 per cent had 4.1-5.0 units; 12.19 per cent had 5.1-6.0 units; and the remaining 5.22 per cent had 6.1 to 7.0 units.

6.1.1.8 *Educational Levels Amongst Men:* The literacy rate amongst men was found to be 70.75 per cent while the remaining *i.e.* 29.25 per cent were illiterates or had zero education. The second category comprising of men who had one to five years of formal education consisted of 31.29 per cent. Those with formal education of six to nine years were placed in the third category *i.e.* 27.89 per cent men belonged here. 11.56 per cent men were placed in the fourth category representing men with formal education of ten to twelve years.

6.1.1.9 *Educational Levels Amongst Women:* The literacy rate of women under study was found to be 31.86 per cent which implies that the remaining 68.14 per cent had zero formal education or were illiterate. Of the remaining 17.04 per cent had received formal education between one to five years; 8.15 per cent had education between ten to 12 years; and 0.74 per cent (1 woman) had received two years of college education.

6.1.1.10 *Combined Literacy Rate of Men and Women:* Was found to be 51.8 per cent

6.1.1.11 *Occupational Patterns of Men:* Of the families under study, 7.82 per cent were unemployed; 16.53 per cent were self-employed; 46.09 per cent were non-govt. employees and 29.56 per cent were govt. employees.

6.1.1.12 *Occupational Patterns of Women:* Of the women under study, 63.48 per cent were housewives; 6.08 per cent were self-employed; and 30.44 per cent were classified as 'employed earning'.

6.1.1.13 *Monthly Per Capita Income:* Was found to be Rs. 148.35 with a standard deviation of Rs. 77.6.

6.1.1.14 *Economic Levels of Families:* The study revealed that there were 27.82 per cent families below 'Poverty Line' *i.e.* with PCI of Rs. 100 or less per month; 19.13 per cent had incomes between Rs. 151-200 per month; 9.56 per cent having incomes between Rs. 201-300; and the remaining 5.22 per cent had income of more than Rs. 301 per month.

6.1.1.15 *Daily Diet Pattern:* There was a long and unhealthy gap of 8 to 10 hours between two major meals in case of all families. Breakfast was dispensed with by 56.53 per cent families and only 43.47 per cent families had it in form of left over roti, bread or biscuit with tea.

Lunch and dinner were taken universally, even if 9.4 per cent families had to beg for it. Lunch usually consisted of *roti* with a curried vegetable and dinner comprised of either *Khichari* or rice and dal at times accompanied by a vegetable. Of the vegetable most commonly reported under 48 hours recall were potatoes, brinjals, cauliflower, tuwar (legume), tomatoes etc. Greens or leafy vegetables though cheap during that season were conspicuous by their absence and same was true of milk products like curds and 'chass'. None reported salads and fruit.

Evening tea could be afforded by only 22.61 per cent and the rest 77.39 per cent did without it. None reported light snacks with tea.

6.1.1.16 *Mean Intake of Essential Food Items Per Day:* Both Per capita intake and per consumption unit intake in the study families were compared against the standard ICMR recommendations of corresponding food items as shown in Table 3.7B. Milk, Rice, Atta (wheat flour in most cases; occasionally bajra). Pulses, Vegetables, Oils/Fats were the daily essentials considered. It was found that daily intake of milk and vegetables (under both categories *viz.* per capita intake and per consumption unit intake) were grossly deficient by the ICMR standards. In case of milk, as against 175 gm. per day per adult, the corresponding means under the two categories were only 52.36 gm. and 63.66 gm respectively. For vegetables as against 180 gm. per day recommended by ICMR, mean per capita intake was 102.71 gm. while the mean per consumption unit intake was slightly higher at 130.64 gm. Under 'cereals' both rice and atta have been considered together by the ICMR and the recommended daily intake is 500 gm. against which the mean per capita intake in our study was 436.0 gm. while the mean per consumption unit intake was 504 gm. or slightly higher than the recommended standard. Similarly in case of pulses, sugar, oil/fats it was found that when mean per consumption unit daily intake was considered against the corresponding standards the situation of study families was quite satisfactory as they were receiving the necessary nutrients in right quantity. Only in case of milk and vegetable consumption there was an alarming nutritional gap.

6.1.1.17 *Incidence of Pregnancy Wastage and Mortality of Underfives:* Less than half *i.e.* 43.48 per cent families exhibited a healthy trend with no incidence of pregnancy waste or underfives' mortality. By implication every second family had experienced loss of one kind or the other. More specifically, 14.78 per cent reported pregnancy wastage; 39.14 per cent reported underfives' mortality; and 2.60 per cent families reported mishaps of both types.

Regarding age at death, it was found that of the total occurence of 66 underfives' deaths, majority *i.e.* 69.70 per cent succumbed below one year while the rest 30.30 per cent died between 1 to 5 years of age. More male children *i.e.* 57.58 per cent as compared to 42.42 per cent female children lost their lives. As per causes of death, though precise data was not available in all cases, the commonest reasons given were diarrhoea, fever and mother's illness etc.

6.1.1.18 *Utilization of Ante-Natal, Natal, Post-Natal and Family Planning Services:* In the study families it was found that only 4.34 per cent women had availed of regular Ante-natal check up as against 93.91 per cent who had not; while 1.73 per cent were sterility or 'not applicable' cases. Here, regular periodicity was defined as at least two check-ups in each trimester. Most women in the present study sought medical advice only in the last three months of pregnancy or the advance stage. This perhaps explained why utilization of Iron supplements, vitamins and Tetanus Toxoid were somewhat better. While 64.34 per cent had taken vitamins and Iron supplements, 33.91 per cent responded in negative and 1.73 per cent were 'n.a.' cases. Regarding Tetanus Toxoid 51.30 per cent responded affirmative; 46.96 per cent in negative, 1.74 per cent being 'n.a.' cases.

To ascertain utilization of natal services, the women were asked to furnish data pertaining to last three or less (in case of lesser children) children born to them. Of the total such 318 births, 43.40 per cent were home deliveries *i.e.* without trained attendance and other natal services and 56.60 per cent were hospital deliveries where professional help was available.

Regarding the customary six-week post-natal examination of mother and child, only 7.83 per cent responded in affirmative and that too because the child had developed some serious health problem. It is surprising that despite more than half the births having occured at hospitals. 90.44 per cent women did not go back for post-natal check up. On the positive side, 58.27 per cent women had followed the medical advice of giving colostrum to the newborn child. Of the remaining 40.0 per cent discarded it while 1.73 per cent were sterile.

Professional advice for spacing births or sterilisation was utilised by 56.52 per cent women while 41.74 per cent utilised neither, the rest 1.73 per cent being 'n.a.' cases. Further query into (permanent only) measures of contraception revealed that a large number *i.e.* 41.73 per cent couples had not undergone either spouse sterilisation. Tubectomy was greatly favoured over Vasectomy; the statistics being 35.65 per cent and 20.0 per cent respectively.

6.1.1.19 *Age at Weaning and Weaning Foods:* The study revealed grossly incorrect weaning practices amongst respondent families. Only 10.44 per cent could be credited for initiating weaning at the correct age of 4 to 6 months. 26.28 per cent can be termed as 'moderately late starters' having begun it when the child was 7 to 9 months old 45.16 per cent formed the modal class where the child was 10 to 14 months old when weaning began.

Amongst 'severely late starters' 8.56 per cent began weaning when the child was 15 to 19 months old; and another 9.56 per cent delayed weaning till the child was 20 to 24 months old.

Mean weaning age was quite high at 11.3 months with the standard deviation of 2.3 months.

The most popular weaning foods were 'rice and dal' or *khichadi*. Many families also give '*roti* with *dal*' or whatever is cooked for the meal. Especially suitable weaning food for infants was reported to be 'glucose biscuits' (?). Few women prepared 'dal soup', 'rice water soup', or fruit juice for infants. Top milk *i.e.* supplementary skimmed buffalo milk or cow's milk was given by a small minority.

6.1.1.20 *Motor and Mental Development Testing of Children between 0-30 months :* Measurements on Bailey's scale (modified by Phatak P. for Indian Children) revealed that there was not a single case of latent disability in the slum families under study.

6.1.2 *Findings Based on Health and Growth-monitoring Intervention for Underfives:* Findings under this sub-head comprise three types. The first category highlights the health status of study children before intervention.

In the second category we include statistical assessment of the seven hypotheses postulated in this regard. And the third category presents findings obtained by multiple regression analysis of three major dependent variables viz. Weight/Height^2 x 100, Haemoglobin status and Nutritional status against relevant predictors *viz.* household size, mother's education per capita monthly income and mother's age.

6.1.2.1 The base-line health status of the underfives study children was very poor. More specifically, mean Wt./Ht.^{2} x 100 ratio in treatment and control groups were .1295 and .1301 respectively as against the standard value of 0.15 for low socio-economic status children; mean haemoglobin levels measured 8.8600 and 8.7160 in treatment and control groups respectively as against the WHO standard of 11.0 gm/dl. for underfives poor children; and lastly a majority of children in both groups belonged to the category of second degree of malnutrition which is defined as the reduction in body weight upto 71-60 per cent of the median weight.

6.1.2.2 Under the impact of the field-experiment, there was an all-round improvement in the treatment group children as shown by the three criteria indicators. More specifically, Wt./Ht.^{2} x100 ratio and haemoglobin level rose to .1441 and 9.4433 respectively while the mean nutritional status moved from second to first degree of malnutrition *i.e.* after intervention it lay between 80-71 per cent of median weight.

6.1.2.1 t-test analysis of means in the case of seven hypotheses postulated in this regard confirmed that the first six hypothesis could be retained at high levels of statistical significance i.e. at $p < .001$ or $p < .05$. The implication here being that the treatment group children recorded significant increase, in their post-intervention measures of weight-for-height, haemoglobin and nutritional status vis-a-vis the respective pre-intervention values. Simultaneously, the 'after only' t-test of treatment and control groups also proved that the treatment group was significantly superior at the end of social intervention. In other words, the health and growth-monitoring interventions under the experiment were impactful in the present context.

6.1.2.2 Hypothesis 7 stating that the incidence of reported morbidity in case of treatment group would be lower than the control group was conclusively rejected on the basis of t-test result. Suitable explanation for this unexpected result have been discussed at length in chapter four, section 4.5.7.1.

6.1.2.3 Multiple regression analysis of predictor variables like household size, mother's age, mother's education and per capita monthly income against criteria variables of weight for height, Haemoglobin and nutritional status revealed that "mother's education" was the single most powerful independent variable which was positively and significantly correlated to all the three dependent variables. R-Square values or the variance produced in each case was high too. Of the remaining variables, household size and mother's age bore a negative correlation but the relationship in none of the three cases was statistically significant. The implication however was that smaller households and younger mothers contributed positively towards health of underfives. Per capita monthly income though positively correlated made no statistically significant impact.

6.1.3 *Findings Based on Health Education Intervention for Mothers*

Findings under this sub-head comprises of two types. The first category includes statistical assessment of the six hypotheses postulated in this regard. In the second category we present findings obtained by multiple regression analysis of aggregate scores of Knowledge, Attitudes and Practices of Health Care of Underfives amongst Mothers as the three major dependent variables against the most relevant predictors, namely, household size, mother's education, per capita monthly income and mother's age.

6.1.3.1 Statistical analysis using t-test in the case of six hypotheses postulated in this context revealed that the former four hypotheses pertaining to change in knowledge and attitudes could be retained at high levels of significance of p-values < .001 or <.05. The implication here being that the treatment group mothers recorded significant increase in their post intervention aggregate scores of knowledge and attitudes vis-a-vis the respective pre-intervention scores. The 'after-only' comparison of knowledge, however, did reveal a slight 'trickle around' spread of knowledge, from the former to the latter group. In the open community setting of the field experiment such sharing of knowledge could not be prevented. But since knowledge gain by control group mothers had increased marginally, it seemed judicious to retain the hypotheses. The two hypotheses on increase in aggregate attitudes score could be retained unambiguously.

6.1.3.2 The last two hypotheses on increase in aggregate practice score could be accepted partially at p<.001 or p<.05 levels of significance. Both hypotheses 12 and 13 contained three sub-hypotheses each in the areas of 'care and management of the sick child'; 'infant feeding' and 'personal hygiene'. t-test analysis of hypotheses 12 revealed that it was tenable with respect to 'care and management of sick child' and 'personal hygiene' but un-tenable in the area of 'infant-feeding' practices. However, in the case of hypotheses 13, it was found to be acceptable only in the area of 'care and management of the sick child' while with respect to practices of 'infant feeding' and 'personal hygiene' it had to be clearly rejected.

6.1.3.3 Multiple Regression analysis between predictor variables like household size, mother's education and per capita monthly income and criteria variables of aggregate scores of knowledge, attitude and practice revealed that as for as aggregate score of knowledge gain was concerned only mother's education was positively and significantly correlated. In the case of aggregate score of attitudes none of the predictor variables had any statistically significant influence whether positive or negative. However, in the case of aggregate score of practice while mother's education was a positive and statistically significant correlate, household size proved to be a negative correlate which was also statistically significant. Contrary to popular belief per capita monthly income was not significantly correlated to any of the three dependent variables. Similarly, mother's age was negatively correlated to all but the relationships were not significant.

6.2 Conclusions

In the light of the summary of major findings, certain conclusions that can be drawn are stated below:

6.2.1 The present intervention module which lay heavy emphasis on multi-disciplinary team approach to improvement of health of underfive slum children was efficient in fulfilling its objectives since the three criteria indicators viz. weight for height measure, haemoglobin status and nutritional status of the treatment group were shown to have increased significantly at the post-intervention stage.

6.2.2 The model has demonstrated how social work profession can assume central responsibility in promoting effective utilisation of resources by the urban poor. On one hand, professional knowledge and skills of a hospital based health care system were provided with the necessary support to out-reach open slums and on the other, the people were made aware of and encouraged to draw benefits from the former. Clearly, this is of much relevance in the context of a developing nation like India, where the resources are scant and the needs are ever increasing.

6.2.3 The module was successful in significantly improving the aggregate scores of knowledge and attitudes regarding health care of underfives amongst the target women *i.e.* there indeed lay positive evidence of cognitive and affective learning by them. However, the module was only partially successful in making a significant impact in the practice area.

In order to explain this un-expected outcome we quote Alleyne *et al.* (1976) who state that behaviour may be inhibited even when knowledge and attitudes are changed because of constraints of conforming with the community, husband rejection, lack of resources, political or religious loyalties in any given cultural context are generation old and the women themselves must feel secure in following time honoured traditions rather than take risks with the new.

At the same time, there is no cause to feel over despondent. According to theories of learning, cognitive and affective type of learning invariably pre-dispose individuals towards behavioural changes or improved psycho-motor functioning. It can be, therefore, suggested here that further interventions with heavier emphasis on improvement of practice would certainly yield the desired results.

6.2.4 Multiple regression analysis finding that mother's education was the single most significant and positive correlate of all the three chosen indicators of child health and aggregate scores of knowledge and practice of health care amongst mothers strongly recommends the need of informal health education interventions of the type incorporated in the present study.

6.2.5 There were several inadvertent or side-gains of the field experiment.

The two, most important ones are mentioned here.

The growth-monitoring interventions and the health education programme in combination raised health-consciousness amongst treatment group mothers. This was reflected in higher reporting of underfives' morbidity by treatment group mothers vis-a-vis the control group at the post intervention stage whereby hypothesis seven had to be rejected. In other words, the treatment group mothers had imbibed the importance of early response to faltering health of their underfive children and report about it.

Secondly, women participants of the health education programme underwent a dramatic change in their total personality. From the stereotype of illiterate, under-priviledged and taciturn women they emerged as bold, relatively well aware and intellectually curious individuals in their own right. Most of our guest speakers were highly impressed by their keen interest in the programme and the quality of questions raised by them.

6.2.6 Finally, in view of the substantial success achieved by the present intervention model in fulfilling most of its stated objectives, its cost-effectiveness and the professional responsibility discharged in the process, it is strongly recommended that such interventions should be replicated under similar conditions. In the next section, we present some 'tested do's' to facilitate future efforts by social work professionals and other practitioners.

6.3 The Emergent Module

The under-lying purpose served by any intervention module is that it facilitates its replication elsewhere under comparable conditions. The emphasis should, however, be on furnishing a set of proven guidelines or experiential lessons and not an supplying ready-to-use programme formats. In fact, it would only be prudent that the future practitioners evolve their own work-plan taking into cognizance, the uniqueness of probable clients, availability of infra-structural devices and the prevailing socio-political environment.

6.3.1 *The Present Field Experiment*: As far as the present field experiment is concerned vivid details have already been presented in chapters one, four and five under various sections *viz.* Research Design; Flow Diagram of the Intervention process; Procedures of Base-Line Survey; Procedures in Application of Input A; Procedures in Application of Input B; *Modus-operandi* of Growth-monitoring and all the section 5.1. What perhaps can be added at this juncture are a few 'useful tips' which emerged directly from our field experience.

6.3.2 *Preparatory Work:* 'Involving the people from the very beginning' is a crucial consequence. While it is true that such projects usually happen at the initiative of community welfare agencies and also that 'health of underfives' is hardly ever a 'felt need' of the community yet the people can be involved in various ways. Door-to-door contacts; seeking leaders' opinion; small group discussions with men and women to explain in simple terms the objectives, expected outcomes, process, approximate intervention period, areas in which community support is needed and clarification of their doubts or apprehensions etc. must precede everything else. Further, no commitment should be made until there is a green signal from the community.

It indeed takes much sensibility, footwork and determined effort to elicit peoples' participation but its a worthy investment all the same. People have some very useful ideas to contribute and they may even volunteer to undertake various responsibilities when we stimulate them appropriately.

Communities often tend to be over-surveyed and sometimes over-intervened these days. it is only proper, therefore, that the interventionists compensate the people for the time and energy which the latter eventually spend on the project. A system of short-term and tangible rewards should be worked out in advance. In the present case, on different occasions biscuits, toffees, handkerchiefs, some plastic items, and a Certificate in Child Health Education were instituted as token incentives for the participant children and their mothers.

Having won the confidence of the people, prepare a tentative outline of the interventive plan in consultation with experts. In a multi-disciplinary situation, it is of fundamental importance that the programme format be thoroughly discussed with other professionals in the team and modified subsequently. Such discussions not only lead to technical refinement of the plan but they also go a long way in developing a healthy team spirit amongst the members and help enrich the resource bank for the project.

Construct, protest and finalise the research tools and measurement scales etc.

Train investigators to upgrade their interviewing skills through field demonstrations and follow up discussions.

Organise training of investigators in administration of Bailey's Developmental Testing Tool. In the present case they were sent to Infant Testing Centre, Faculty of Home Science, M.S. University of Baroda.

Locate community resources to finance the cost of medicines and honorarium of the CHV.

The agency may have adequate manpower but engaging a volunteer from amongst the people themselves helps increase their faith in the project. Besides, it is a practical arrangement wherein the interventionist is in a position to maintain a live, two-way contact with the community.

Prepare well in advance, forms for medical examination; register for recommended treatment and referrals; morbidity record register; height, weight and haemoglobin record register; registration cards assigning identification numbers to each child; and physical lay-out of furniture and other equipment required for various events.

Procure in time medicine for deworming treatment (Mebendezol), Vitamin pills, iron pills, paediatric syrups, raod-to-health cards for growth-monitoring and audio-visuals aids for the health education programme.

Intervention Phase

Day and time for health education sessions, and other planned activities should be decided in consultation with the women. Otherwise, the interventionist would not know about the ration collection day, local social calender and festivals when women observe fast etc. Obviously, scheduling of project activities on such inconvenient days could evoke a negative response.

Further, organisation and co-ordination during each event must be very strong *i.e.* as far as possible, there should be no delays or postponements; equipment snags; communication gaps amongst professionals as well as between the people and the project team; and lack of role clarity at any level. Much effort is required to ensure all this but it helps build peoples' confidence.

The project team must critically evaluate each component activity at the end, amongst themselves. Such exercises are necessary to assess strengths and short-comings of the work done and aid in improving the quality of future programmes.

Demonstration of high work-discipline, sincerity and efficient time management by the interventionists begets them respect as professionals and affection as individuals. Consequently their (peoples') enthusiasm and co-operation towards the project grows.

So far it has been emphasized how vitally important it is to work as per a carefully planned schedule. At the same time, interventionist must recognise certain exigencies from the peoples' view point and be accommodating about them, no matter how trivial or inconsequential the situation may seem to the former.

Post Intervention Phase

Formal and Informal vote of thanks must be extended to people, collaborating professionals and several others who contributed in numerous small ways.

Goodwill earned through the course of one project must be masterfully used to advantage for planning of future interventions with the people. Indeed, this to some extent would depend on the agency policy and programmes.

Follow-up action as indicated by the major findings and outcomes must be pursued in right earnest. For as Park and Park (1985) have put it:

> Few people can learn all that is new in a single period. Repetition at intervals is extremely useful. It assists comprehension and understanding. Every health campaign needs re-inforcement; we may call it a booster dose.

APPENDICES

APPENDIX 'A'

FATEHGUNJ SAMAJ KALYAN KENDRA, FACULTY OF SOCIAL WORK M.S. UNIVERSITY OF BARODA

Base-Line Survey of Socio-economic Status: Health and Nutrition of 0-5 year Old Children from a slum Community

Interview No

Date: Time:

A. *Identification and Socio-Cultural Data:*

Name of HOH:

Name of LOH:

Postal Address:

Religion:

Caste:

Mother Tongue:

Native Place:

Year of Migration:

Year of stay at:

Present Address

B. *Family Information:*

Sr No	Name of family members	Relation-ship to HOH	Age & Date of Birth & immu. sta-tus in the case of 0-5	Educa-tion	Occup-ation	Monthly Income	Special * health condition if any (write).
1	2	3	4	5	6	7	8

* Pregnancy, Nursing mother, handicapped child, chronically ill person (Name disease).

C. *Compute and Record:*

Number of family members in the dwelling unit	:
Total family monthly Income	:
Per Capita Monthly Income	:
No of 0-5 year olds	:
15 to 44 years old women	: Pregnant/Lactating/No special condition

D. *Economic condition*	:
(a) *Indebtedness*	: Yes/No
If Yes, Amount	:
Source	:
Rate of interest	:
Period of repayment	:
Instalments, if any	:
(b) *Savings*	: Yes/No
If yes, how much per month?	: ....

Investment in cash amount, from interest earned etc.

(c) *Assets:*

(i) House	(vi) Furniture items
(ii) Cattle	(vii) Radio/Transistor
(iii) Land	(viii) Tape recorder
(iv) Cycle	(ix) T.V. Set.
(v) Rickshaw or any other vehicle	(x) Any other

E. *Housing and Environment**

* Data to be collected by observation and secondary methods

Area: Less than 250 sq. ft	Rented/Owned
– 250 + to 500 sq. ft	Kutcha/Semi Pucca/Pucca
– 500 to 750 sq. ft	

Public utilities available:

Drinking water	— Distance from house
Electricity in the dwelling	— Yes/No
Latrine	— Yes/No/Public
Drainage	— Yes/No
Ventilation	— Poor/Good
Surrounding environment	— Poor/Good
Garbage disposal	— Available/Not available

F. *Health and Nutrition data Pertaining to the Family as a whole.*

(a) Normal meal pattern
Meal with time

(b) Actual food taken in the past 48 to 72 hours.

Day & Time	Meal	Items	Ingred	Quantity in Gms

(c) Daily consumption of the following:

(i) Milk ____________ Gms.
(ii) Rice ____________ Cups. (Standard cup size to ____________ be shown to respondent.)
(iii) Vegetable ____________ Gms.
(iv) Atta ____________ Cups.
State type: Jowar
Bajra
Chana mixed
Soya mixed
Wheat
Any other
(v) Pulses ____________ Cups.
(vi) Fruit: ____________

(d) Monthly consumption of the following:

(i) Sugar ____________ kg.
(ii) Cooking oil ____________ kg.
(iii) Fuel ____________ ltr.
(iv) Rice ____________ kg.
(v) Pulses ____________ kg.
(vi) Atta ____________ kg.
(vii) Non-Veg. item ____________
(viii) Eggs

(e) Did any family member suffer any serious illness in the past 5 years?

Sr No.	Name	Age	Disease	Whether/Died Disabled/ Cured?	Remarks Trt. Continues or not?
1	2	3	4	5	6
1.					
2.					
3.					
4.					
5.					
6.					

(f) Normal pattern of Health Services Sought:
Normally, whenever there is anyone sick in the family do you visit:

(i) Bhuva
(ii) Allopath (Private Practitioner)
(iii) Allopath (Free Govt/BMC Services ESI/CGHS)
(iv) Homeopath
(v) Ayurvedic Doctor
(vi) Any other
Instruction: Ask for any old prescription note.

(g) How much approx per month do you spend on medicines

(h) Do you spend for curative service alone? Yes/No
if no, then on what other tonics (promotional)
do you spend?...
How much.....

(i) Family Planning:
Have you adopted Family Planning? Yes/No
Measures: Temporary Permanent
1.
2.
3.

(j) Child Mortality (0 to 5 year olds)
No. of children in the family:

	Male	Female
In the beginning :		
At present :		
Age of death :		
Reason for death :		
Year of death :		

(k) No. of children born at home...

No. of children born at hospital...

(l) Whether supplementary foods are given to infants and pre-schoolers?

Stage	Food given	Age at which started (Weaning Age)	Reasons for given foods
Infant			
(0-1)			
1.			
2.			
3.			
Pre-schooler			
(1-5)			
1.			
2.			
3.			

(m) In the case of pregnant mothers

1. Order of pregnancy-
2. Sources of ante-natal care
   1. Nil
   2. Trained dai
   3. Untrained dai
   4. Hospital (Govt)
   5. Dispensary (Govt)
   6. Qualified private practitioner
   7. Unqualified practitioner
   8. Relative/neighbours
   9. Any other

(n) Whether takes any folic tablets at present or had taken earlier during pregnancy Yes/No

(o) Tetanus Toxiod.

1. Not taken
2. Received one dose
3. Received two doses

(p) How often do you visit ante-natal clinic?....

(q) Post-natal Care

1. After delivery, did you seek medical care for your self and the infant? Yes/No

If yes, when and for what? ____________________________

____

If no, why? ____________________________

____

2. In case of hospital delivery, were you advised about any of the following by doctors?

(i) Giving Colostrum to the infant Yes/No
If yes, did you do it?.......

(ii) Nutritious diet for health of Mother and Infant? Yes/No
If yes, did you follow the advice?

(iii) Spacing and Family Planning? Yes/No
If yes, did you heed the advice?

(G) *Bailey's Test for Motor and Mental Development of Children between 0-30 months (to detect hidden disability)*

Ist Month

a. Limb thrust in play
b. Lateral head movements
c. Stares for a while

2nd Month

a. Responses to rattling sound
b. Follows movements around
c. Observes surroundings by moving head and eyes.

3rd Month

a. Horizontal eye co-ordination: Red ring
b. Responds to voice
c. Lifts head at the shoulder

4th Month

a. Holds head steady
b. Recognises mother
c. Dorsal suspension lifts head

5th Month

a. Tries to grasp moving objects
b. Develops hand grip
c. Sits for a while with support

6th Month

a. Rolls from back to stomach
b. Follows sound
c. Likes to play with paper

7th Month

a. Notices presence of unknown persons. reacts by crying or becoming quiet.

b. Pulls to sitting position

8th Month

a. Likes to throw things
b. Sits without support for a while

9th Month

a. Sits already and looks around
b. Can hold things in both hands
c. Playful response to mirror
d. Pulls to standing position

10th Month

a. Pulls string: Secures ring
b. Likes frolic play
c. Makes crawling movement

11th Month

a. Rings bell purposefully
b. Scoops pellet
c. Sits along with good coordination
d. Stands up by furniture

12th Month

a. Can identify objects
b. Says dada or equivalent

12th and 15th Month

a. Walks with support
b. Claps hands
c. Responds to negative commands
d. Turns pages of book

15th to 18th Month

a. Stands without support
b. Speaks monosyllable words
c. Attempts to scribble
d. Can throw a ball
e. Can stand on his own
f. Walks without support
g. Uses gestures to make wants known.

18th to 24th Month

a. Shows shoes, other clothing or own toy
b. Uses expressive jargon
c. Can ascend and descend stairs with help
d. Expresses needs by speaking

24th to 30 month

a. Speaks sentences of two-three words
b. Names two-three objects
c. Can ascend and descend stairs without support
d. Stands on one foot for a while.

APPENDIX 'B'

Interview Schedule of Knowledge, Attitude and Practice about Health Care Amongst the mothers of (0-5) years olds in a slums community—

Part-I Identification Data and Practice Component

Notes

1: Identification data of the child is very essential as with the help of it the practice carried out by the mothers of 0-5 year olds according to their surroundings can be related.

2: This section includes two divisions. One consists of questions regarding identification data of the child.

3: The other section includes questions which are related to the practices carried out by the mothers in the areas of personal hygiene which are taken during common diseases and diet of the child.

Interview No. Time:

Date:

(A) *Identification Data*

1. Names of the children: (i) (ii) (iii)
2. Sex of the Children: (i) (ii) (iii)
3. Name of the mother:

(B)

Sr. No.	Name of the Family members	Relation to HOH	Age	Education	Occupation	Monthly Income
1.						
2.						
3.						
4.						
5.						
6.						
7.						

(C) *Compute and Record*

No. of family members :
Total family monthly income :
Per Capita monthly income :
Mother:

Pregnant:
Lactating:
Health condition:

Practice of Personal Hygiene by Mothers.

1. How many times a day does you child brush teeth?
   Once/twice/irregular
2. What do you use for brushing teeth?
   Tooth paste/Neem/Salt/Tooth powder/Home made tooth powder/any other.
3. In schools children play together and remain in contact with each other for a long period so there is a greater scope for infection of Lice and dandruff. What is your opinion?......
4. Does your child have Lice or dandruff? Yes/No
5. If yes then what do you do to remove them?
   1. Tells them to remove
   2. Mother removes it by hand
   3. Kerosene treatment
   4. D.D.T.
   5. Fine Comb
   6. Napthalene balls
   7. Any others
6. How many times the hair is washed in a week?
   Once/Twice/More/Every day
7. Since last two years Gujarat has had a severe water scarcity. Under such circumstances what type of problems does your family face?......
8. Are you able to give bath to your child daily? Yes/No
9. Which of the following do you use during bath?
   Soap/Besan/Pumice Stone/none of the above.
10. Personal hygiene status of the mother to be recorded by observation by the investigator.

Information	Pre Record	Post Record
Nails		
Hair		
Clothing		
General Appearance		

11. Generally children don't like to wear clothes in summer seasons: Comments........
12. Does your child act in same day? Yes/No
13. How many times a day do you change his/her clothes? Once/Twice

Care taken during common diseases

1. What kind of treatment do you seek for the common diseases?
   (i) Homeopathy
   (ii) Allopathy
   (iii) Ayurvedic
   (iv) Home Remedies
   (v) Any other
2. Do you give medicines as per doctor's instructions?
   Yes/No
   If no, why?......
3. What do you do when the child refuses to take medicines?
   Force him
   Do not force him
   Make it in powder forms
   Sweeten it
   Any other.
4. When you consult any doctor then he prescribes a complete course of medicines for cure. Do you take medicines till the course is completed or do you stop when the child gets well?.....

Diet and Nutrition

1. In your daily cooking whose choice of food do you consider often?

	Pre	Post
Husband's		
Son's		
Daughter's		
Your own		
No particular		

2. Does your child like some special item?
   Pre ....
   Post ....

If yes, What?

Pre ....

Post ....

3. How often do you prepare it?

Pre ....

Post ....

Part-II Composite Component

Notes 1: This section includes such items of inquiry which have more than one relevant component of study, namely, Knowledge (K), Attitude (A), Practice (P). Example of such items are breast feeding, weaning family planning etc.

2. Questions pertaining to each sub-division K, A or P have been arranged in one single block in such a way as to ensure a logical sequence. However each question bears a code of K/A/P to facilitate data analysis at a later stage.
3. The investigator should proceed with the question as per the serial number prefixed.

Breast Feeding

1- A According to you, is breast-feeding important for infant health?

Yes/No

Pre

Post

2-K What exactly are the merits of breast-feeding?

	Mentioned	Not mentioned
(i) It is a complete food for newborn		
Pre		
Post		
(ii) The practice helps in spacing children		
Pre		
Post		
(iii) Provides love, warmth and emotional security.		
Pre		
Post		
(iv) Very Convenient		
Pre		
Post		
(v) Helps uterus contract back to its normal size		

Pre

Post

(vi) Any other

Pre

Post

3-P Did you breast-feed your children? Yes/No

If yes, how long?.......

If no, why?......

4-P In some communities, collostrum is considered impure and therefore discarded. In your case, what did you do?.......

If given, why?.......

If discarded, why?......

5-K What do you know about Collostrum?

(i) It is a thick, yellowish secretion for 48 hours immediately after delivery

	Mentioned	Not mentioned
Pre		
Post		

(ii) Provides life-long immunity against some diseases

Pre

Post

6-A According to you how should the child be fed?

(i) As and when child demands?

	Mentioned	Not mentioned
Pre		
Post		

(ii) Whenever the child cries.

Pre

Post

(iii) At Fixed intervals

Pre

Post

(iv) Every 2/3/4/5 hours

Pre

Post

Weaning

1-K A child for his/her growth does not need solid foods till he/she asks for them

True	False
Pre	
Post	

2- P In your case, at which age did you start your child on solids?
Youngest Child......
Second Youngest Child......
Third Youngest Child.....

3-P Which solid foods did you give your children for weaning purpose?......

4-K Which common weaning foods would you advise a new mother to give to her child

		Mentioned	Not mentioned
(i)	Khichadi	Pre	
		Post	
(ii)	Banana	Pre	
		Post	
(iii)	Roti mashed with dal	Pre	
		Post	
(iv)	Bread with milk/tea	Pre	
		Post	
(v)	Rice Water	Pre	
		Post	
(vi)	Boiled Vegetable	Pre	
		Post	
(vii)	Biscuits	Pre	
		Post	
(viii)	Milk and rice	Pre	
		Post	
(ix)	Dal soup	Pre	
		Post	
(x)	Any other	Pre	
		Post	

5-ABy breast feeding the child as long as possible as without starting him on solid foods, a mother can ensure that—

(i) The child does not pass stools often

	True	False
Pre		
Post		

(ii) The child grows to be fat and healthy

	True	False
Pre		
Post		

Family Planning

1-K In our country, through mass media, there is extensive propoganda about family planning for the past 25 years or so. In your opinion there are any advantages of family planning

	Yes	No
Pre		
Post		

If yes, mention them

		Mentioned	Not mentioned
(i) Better health of mother	Pre		
	Post		
(ii) Better health of children	Pre		
	Post		
(iii) Due to small family size purchasing power increases	Pre		
	Post		
(iv) The family can spend more on education	Pre		
	Post		
(v) The family can spend more on food	Pre		
	Post		
(vi) The family can spend more on housing and clothing etc	Pre		
	Post		
(vii) The parents can give more attention and time to children	Pre		
	Post		
(viii) Any other	Pre		
	Post		

2-K In this context does the nation benefit in any way.

	Yes	No
Pre		
Post		

If yes, how?

Pre ....

Post ....

3-K By the way, which are the major social problems this country is facing today?

Pre ....

Post ....

4-K Now we come back to you and your family in particular.

Please give your opinion on few statements below.

(i)-A. In our Hindu/Christian/Muslim religion and culture it is usually said that children are a gift of god and we should not interfere with what the god wants for us.

	Pre	Post
Strongly agree		
agree		
Neutral		
Strongly disagree		
disagree		

(ii)-A. Some people say, there should be preferably two sons in each family

	Pre	Post
Strongly agree		
agree		
Neutral		
Strongly disagree		
disagree		

(iii)-A. In any case, there should be at least one son in each family

	Pre	Post
Strongly agree		
agree		
Neutral		
Strongly disagree		
disagree		

(iv)-A. Hypothetically, what is the maximum number of children that you would have to get a son?

Pre ....

Post ....

(v)-A. Again, hypothetically speaking, in case of miscarriages, how many pregnancies would you be prepared to undergo to get a son?

Pre ....

Post ....

(vi)-A. Daughters are a burden or liability.

	Pre	Post
Strongly agree		
agree		
Neutral		
Strongly disagree		
disagree		

(vii)-A. On the whole, do you favour or disfavour large family? (of four or more living children)

	Pre	Post
Favours		
Neutral		
Disfavours		

5-K What methods of contraception have you heard of?

	Pre	Post
(i) Natural		
(ii) Rhythm		
(iii) Oral pills		
(iv) Copper T		
(v) Diaphragm		
(vi) Vasectomy		
(vii) Tubectomy/Laparoscopy		
(viii) Nirodh		

6-P. Have you ever practiced any of these methods so far? Yes/No
If yes, why? ....
If no, why? ....

7-P. Did you experience any side effects? .... Yes/No
If yes, what? ....

8-P. From your relatives and family friends have you known of any person who has suffered side effects of family planning measures?
Yes/No
If yes, details.......... ....
....
....

Pre-Natal Care

1-P. Pregnancy is a natural condition in a woman's life cycle. But there is a diverse opinion on the religious, social and management practices during this period. As we are talking about child health, in your community is a woman encouraged to seek medical advice after conception?

2-P. In your case did you consult a doctor? Yes/No
If yes, when? ....
If no, why? ....

3-P. What advice/treatment did the doctor prescribe for you?........
Did you fully carry out doctor's advice or did you face any difficulty,

in following it completely?.........

4-K. Which vaccine is given to the mother during pregnancy?

	Mentioned	Not mentioned
(i) Tetanus Toxoid	Pre	
	Post	
(ii) When is it given? Between 16 to 36 weeks		
	Pre	
	Post	
(iii) How many doses are given?		
	Pre	
	Post	

5-K. Does the mother need to take any supplementary tonics/tablets in this condition Yes/No

Pre

Post

6-K. If yes, please mention which

	Mentioned	Not mentioned
(i) Iron	Pre	
	Post	
(ii) Calcium	Pre	
	Post	
(iii) Protein	Pre	
	Post	

7-K. What advice would you give to a primi-para mother?
Mark if mentioned and X if not mentioned

	Pre	Post
(i) Consult a doctor and follow his advice.		
(ii) In case of a normal pregnancy take regular light exercise		
(iii) Continue routine household work		
(iv) Get more nutrition in daily diet		
(v) Relax physically and mentally and think of pleasant things		
(vi) Eat for two		
(vii) Any other		

Post Natal Care

1-P. Did you consult a doctor immediately after delivery in case of home delivery. Yes/No

If yes, when? ....

If no, why? ....

2-P. Did you consult a doctor after your return home in case of a hospital delivery Yes/No
If yes, when? ....
If no, why? ....

3-P. Were you advised about family planning measures at this juncture by a medical or para-medical worker Yes/No
If yes, did you follow the advice?.......

4-K. What do you know about post-natal care in the context of mother and child health
Pre ....
Post ....

Immunization

1-K. What are the different vaccines recommended for 0-5 year olds? Mark if mentioned and X if not mentioned

	Pre	Post
B.C.G.		
Triple/D.P.T.		
Polio		
Measles		

2-K. What do you know about the schedule (timing) of immunization? (investigator should inquire about the items as mentioned in the top box in the following table.)

Vaccine	Time of Measure-ment	Which disease is protected against?	Oral Vaccine or Injectable?	No of doses	Age at which the dose are given
B.C.G.	Pre				
	Post				
D.P.T.	Pre	(i)			First dose ....
		(ii)			Second dose ....
		(iii)			Third dose ....
	Post	(i)			First dose ....
		(ii)			Second dose ....
		(iii)			Third dose ....
Polio	Pre				First dose ....
					Second dose ....
					Third dose ....
	Post				First dose ....
					Second dose ....
					Third dose ....

Measles	Pre
	Post
D.P.T.Booster	Pre
	Post
Polio Booster	Pre
	Post

3-P. Are your underfives immunised in time? Yes/No
If yes, completely/Partially? First underfive:
(Record the investigator's assessment Second underfive:
separately for each target child) Third underfive:
If no, why? ....

4-P. Where did you go for immunization?
(i) S.S.G. Hospital
(ii) Any other Hospital
(iii) Neighboured Vaccination Centre
(iv) Anganwadi Pensionpura
(v) M.C.H. Centre, Fatehgunj
(vi) Any other

Part-III

Notes : 1 Knowledge about the disease management and its harmful effects are based on the individual experiences and practices generally carried out by the mothers.

2 The section includes questions regarding the knowledge of the mothers about symptoms; complications; harmful effects; disease management and prevention of the common diseases.

3 In our pretesting we included thirteen common diseases namely Polio, Measles, Chicken Pox, Cholera, Malaria, Diarrhoea, Tuberculosis, Anaemia, Scabies, Whooping Cough, Common Cold, Tetanus and Diphtheria. However, we found sufficient knowledge among the mothers regarding some diseases and therefore, dropped the same from the final list of diseases which is as per below:
Measles, Chicken Pox, Tetanus, Diarrhoea, Scabies and Anaemia.

4 Mark if the listed response is given to the underlined questions under each disease and mark X if the listed items are not mentioned.

1. Name of the Disease: Chicken Pox Pre Post
Gujarati Name: Achhabada

1. *Usual season of occurrence?*
   (i) Winter months

2. *Symptoms?*
   (i) Cold anorexia (loss of appetite)
   (ii) Mild fever
   (iii) Malaise (feeling of general discomfort)
   (iv) Rash remains for longer period
   (v) Eruption of papular rash over the child's trunk and unexposed parts of body and later on exposed parts such as face and even in mouth.
   (vi) Child is covered with all stages of rash so that crusts, vesicles and papules are all evident at the same time. Child runs a fever corresponding in intensity with severity of the infection.

3. *Complications and Harmful Effects?*
   (i) Unfortunate site of a vesicle such as the child's cornea which may result in a corneal scar or to encephalitis (inflammation of brain), it may effect eyes of the child.

4. *Disease Management?*
   (i) Seeking medical treatment
   (ii) Cold foods and liquids, anti fever/Antipyeritic medication to reduce child's discomfort
   (iii) Keep the child's nails cut short to prevent the child from scratching his lesions.
   (iv) If possible cover his hands with socks securely tied around his wrists.
   (v) Calamine lotion or a specific bath for several times a day can be applied.

5. *Prevention?*
   (i) The child should be isolated from other children in order to prevent further spread of the disease.

Name of the disease: Measles Pre Post
Gujarati Name: Ori

1. *Usual seasons of occurrence*
   (i) Late Winter
   (ii) Early spring

2. *Symptoms?*
   (i) Hyperirritability
   (ii) Cold and Running nose
   (iii) Fever

(iv) Conjunctivitis (Inflammation of eyes)
(v) Cold photophobia (Child fears direct light)
(vi) Anorexia (loss of appetite)
(vii) Rapidly spreading rash on entire body (14 days after initial contact)
(viii) High fever and malaise (feeling of discomfort)

3. *Complications and Harmful Effects?*
(i) Pneumonia
(ii) Meningitis
(iii) Encephalitis (Inflammation of brain)
(iv) Disease could be fatal in some cases.

4. *Disease Management?*
(i) Isolation of the infected child
(ii) Seeking medical treatment
(iii) Special care of mal-nourished child
(iv) Bland food

5. *Prevention?*
(i) Isolate the child to prevent exposing more children to infection.
(ii) Soft and shaded light in child's room in order to protect his eyes from a residual light sensitivity
(iii) Complete bed-rest to prevent all complications.
(iv) Immunization of child during the period of 9 months to one year.

Name of the Disease: Anaemia Pre Post

1. *Usual seasons of occurrence*
(i) No particular season

2. *Symptoms?*
(i) Pallor (Paleness)
(ii) Swelling of Face
(iii) Fatigue
(iv) Weakness
(v) White and pale skin
(vi) Pale and whitish nails
(vii) Pale and whitish tongue and eyes
(viii) Nails become flat or concave, depressed or spoon shaped
(ix) Not gaining height and weight

3. *Complications and Harmful Effects?*
(i) Respiratory Difficulty
(ii) Headache
(iii) Dimness of vision
(iv) Faintness

4. *Disease Management?*
   (i) Iron rich diet
   (ii) Green Vegetables, Eggs, Carrots during season pumpkin, papaya.

1. Name of the Disease: Diarrhoea
   Gujarati Name: Jada
   Pre Post

1. *Usual season of occurrence*
   (i) No particular season
2. *Symptoms?*
   (i) Soft pale, bulky, foul smelling stools
   (ii) Loss of appetite
   (iii) Becomes irritable
   (iv) Change in moods from reserved to aggressive
   (v) Vomitting
3. *Disease Management?*
   (i) Low fat, high protein and simple carbohydrate diet.
   (ii) According to the response to the treatment increase in variety of food
   (iii) To give light food till the symptoms disappear
   (iv) O R T (Oral Rehydration Therapy)
4. *Complications and Harmful Effects?*
   (i) Dehydration
   (ii) Can be fatal
5. *Prevention?*
   (i) Improving Dietary habits.
   (ii) Improving personal hygiene of child and mother.

Name of the disease: Tetanus Pre Post

1. *Usual seasons of occurrence*
   (i) 5 to 14 days after accident, Cut etc.
2. *Symptoms?*
   (i) Fever
   (ii) Aches and pains
   (iii) Stiffness of muscles especially the mouth and jaws
   (iv) Inability to open mouth or to swallow
   (v) Hyperirritability and restlessness
   (vi) Muscles spasms
   (vii) Headaches
3. *Complications and Harmful Effects?*
   (i) Convulsions may cause the child's death (absence of oxygen)
   (ii) Could be fatal

4. *Disease Management?*
   (i) Adequate cleansing of the wound with soap and water helps to reduce the possibility of developing infection
   (ii) Special care of malnourished child to avoid further complications
   (iii) Seeking medical treatment

5. *Prevention?*
   (i) Immunization of child
   (ii) 3 Successive injections of tetanus toxoid at 4th month
   5th month 6th month
   (iii) Booster doses at 18 months
   5 years
   12 years
   (iv) Isolation of the infected child and his equipment to preve..t the spread of infections.

Scabies

1. *Usual seasons of occurrence?* Pre Post
   (i) More common during winters

2. *Symptoms?*
   (i) Severe itching which is worse at night
   (ii) This Rash on wrists, elbows, around nipples, umbilian lower abdomen, genitals, thigh, legs.

3. *Disease Management?*
   i) All the family members should be treated at the same time. The clothes, bed linen and towels should be boiled and ironed.

4. *Prevention?*
   The patient must be bathed and scrub the body to lay open the burrows. After the bath the skin is dried and apply medication on the whole body as advised by doctors.

Attitude Component

Notes: 1. Attitudes are usually formed on the basis of traditional practices, beliefs or individual experiences.
2. The section of the interview schedule restricts itself to attitudes of mothers which affect their utilization of health services relevant to growth and development of 0-5 years old.
3. With regard to question numbered three the respondent may be asked to opine only if she came in contact with the hospital system or the type of personnel mentioned.

1. Government of India studies in different parts of the country show that the number of boys brought for medical treatment far outnumber girls. Similar is the situation in the case of adult men and women with regard to health services utilised by them. Based on your experience what reasons can you assign for the prevailing situation?

Pre ....

....

Post ....

....

2. Government statistics also show that life expectancy amongst women is much lower than men. Again, what could be the reasons for this, according to you?

Pre ....

....

Post ....

....

3. You must have come in contact with the hospital staff such as Doctors, Nurses and Social workers etc. when some family member, relative or neighbour was hospitalised,. On majority of occasions, what was you experience of the following:

	Co-operative	Non-Co-operative
Doctors		
Nurses		
Social Workers		
Family Planning workers		
Medicine Suppliers		
Vaccinators		

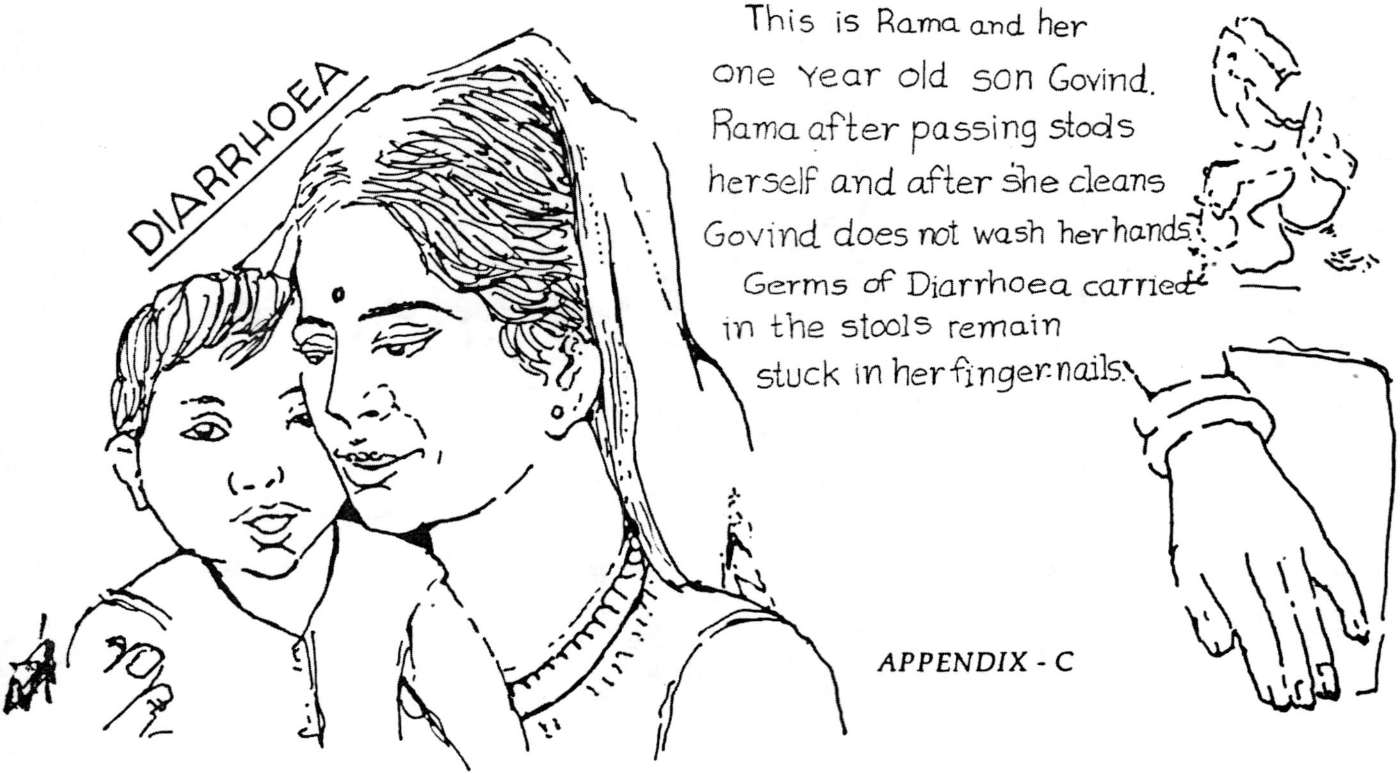
DIARRHOEA
This is Rama and her
one Year old son Govind.
Rama after passing stools
herself and after she cleans
Govind does not wash her hands.
Germs of Diarrhoea carried
in the stools remain
stuck in her finger-nails.

APPENDIX - C

APPENDIX - C (contd.)

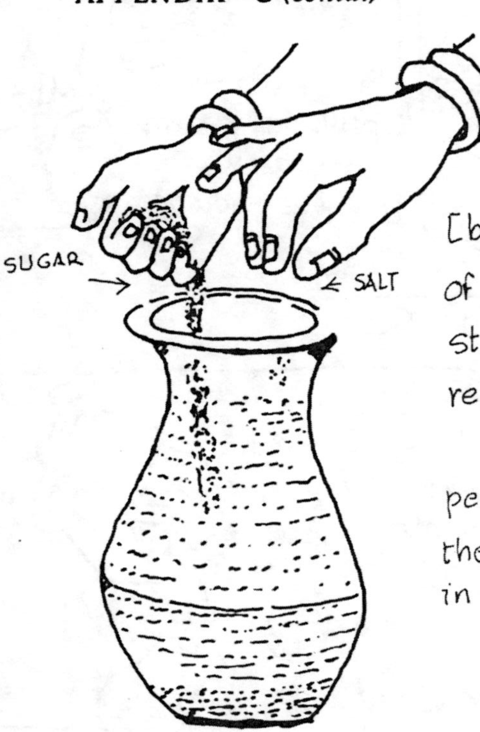

To prevent the child's diarrhoes from taking a serious turn give him lime juice with salt & Sugar frequently. How would you prepare this lime juice? Take 500 ml. of [boiled and cooled] water. Add of fistfuls of sugar and 2 pinches of salt and stir to dissolve. Give this mixture repeatedly to the child during the day.

At least give 6 to 7 glasses per day to the child, This replaces the loss of water & minerals in body caused by diarrohea

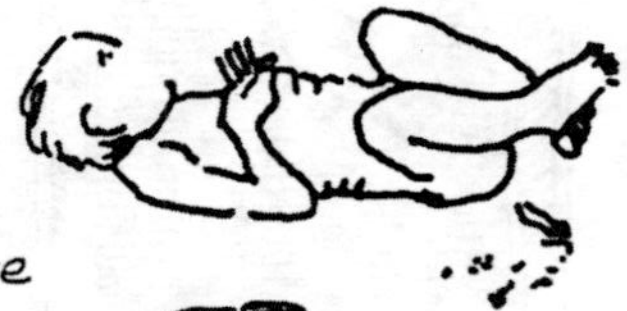

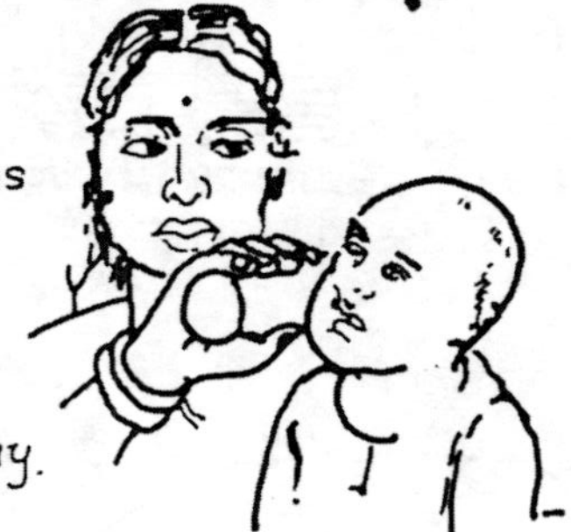

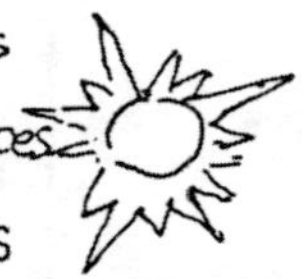

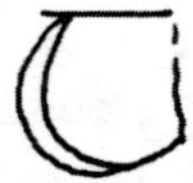

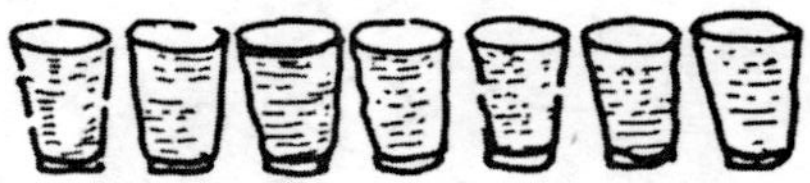

APPENDIX - C (contd.)

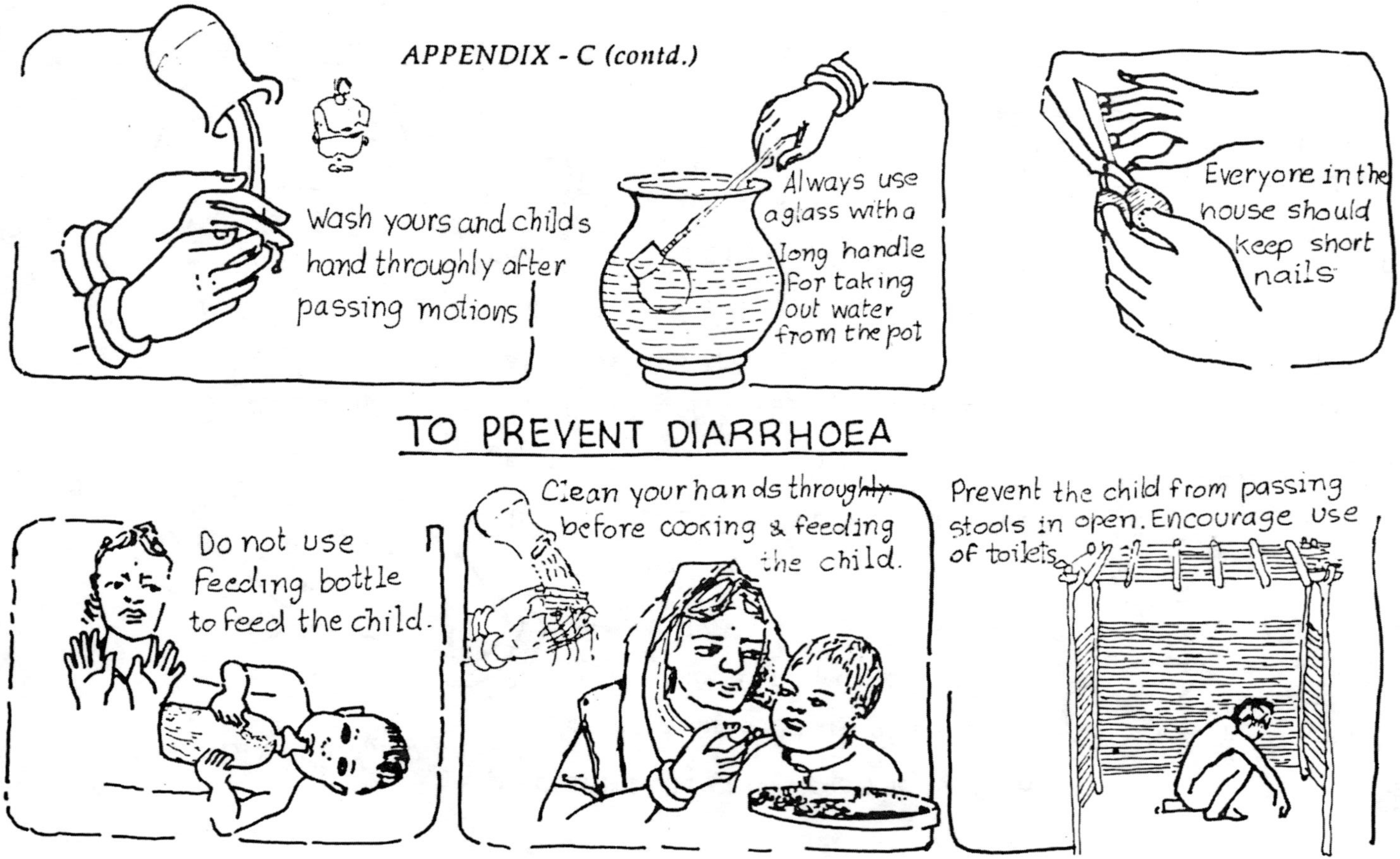

Young Children lose a lot of body weight due to repeated motions. He becomes prone to illness.

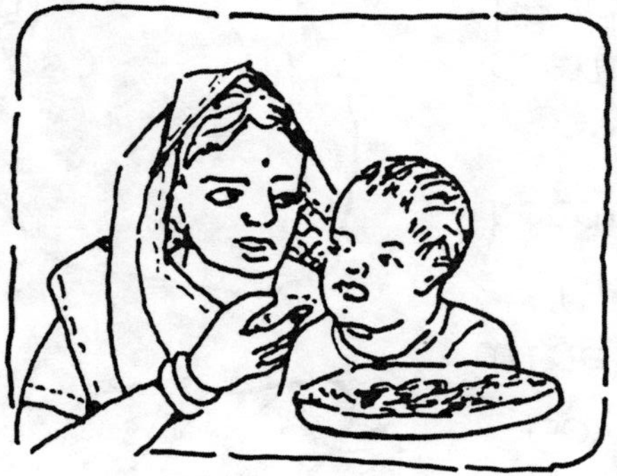

Feed the child everything that is cooked at home.

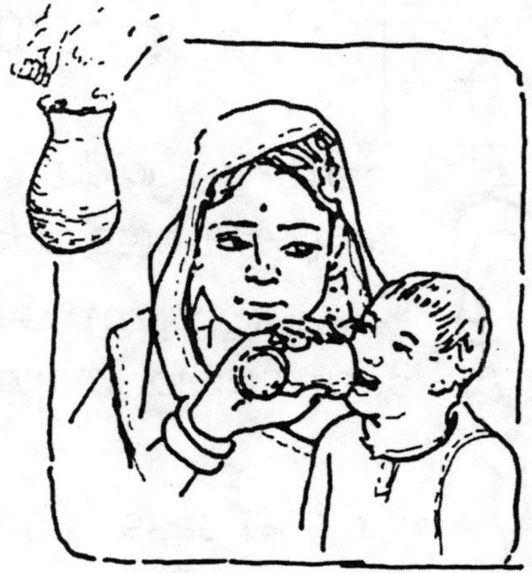

Give him lime juice with salt & sugar Frequently when he is down with diarrhoea.

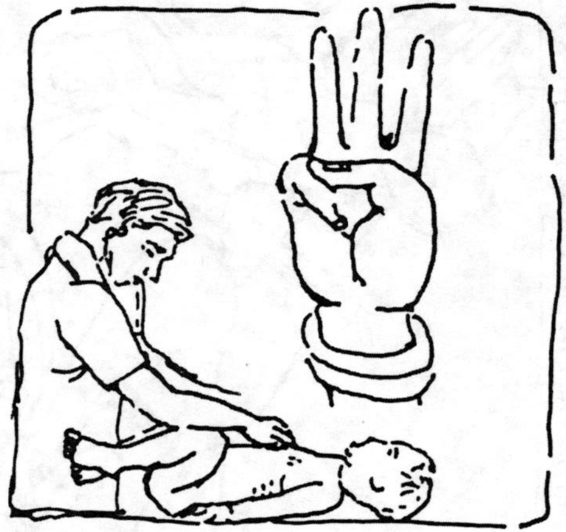

If the motions do not come under control within 2 or 3 days take the child to a doctor.

APPENDIX - C (contd.)

APPENDIX - C (contd.)

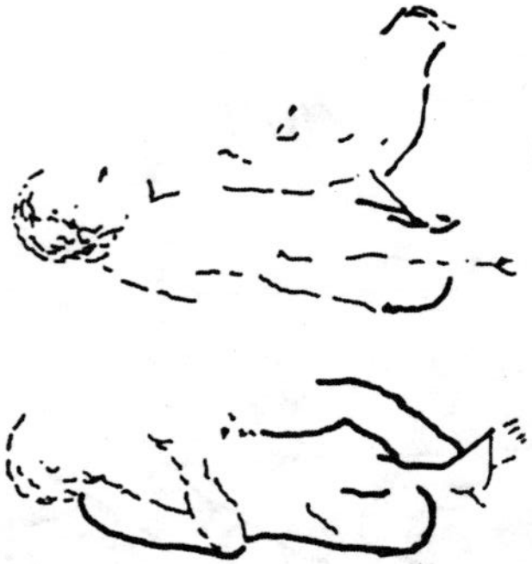

The skin of Govind's stomach loses elasticity. It takes time for the skin to restore back to normalcy.

Govind passes lesser urine.

The colour of his urine becomes dark yellow.

A depression can be seen on top of Govind's head

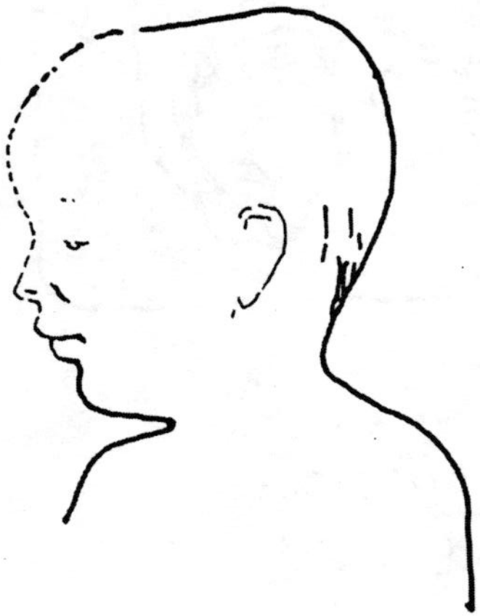

GOVIND DIES

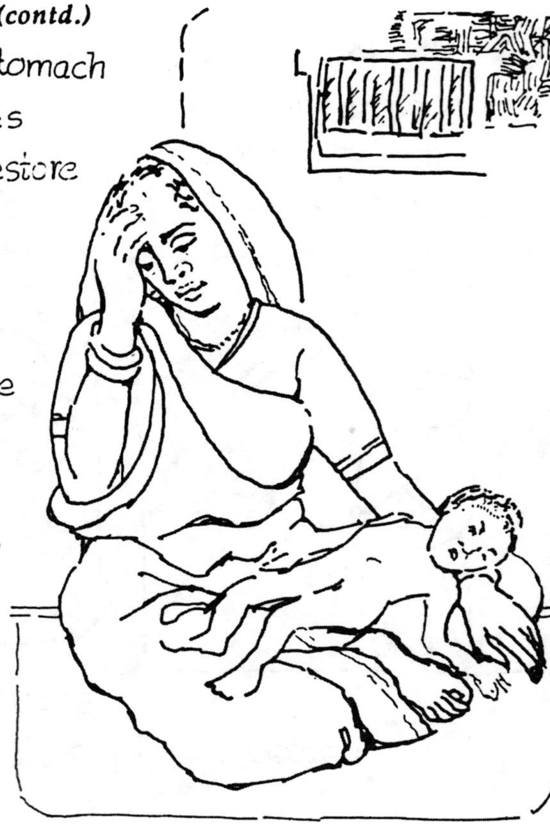

APPENDIX - C (*contd.*)

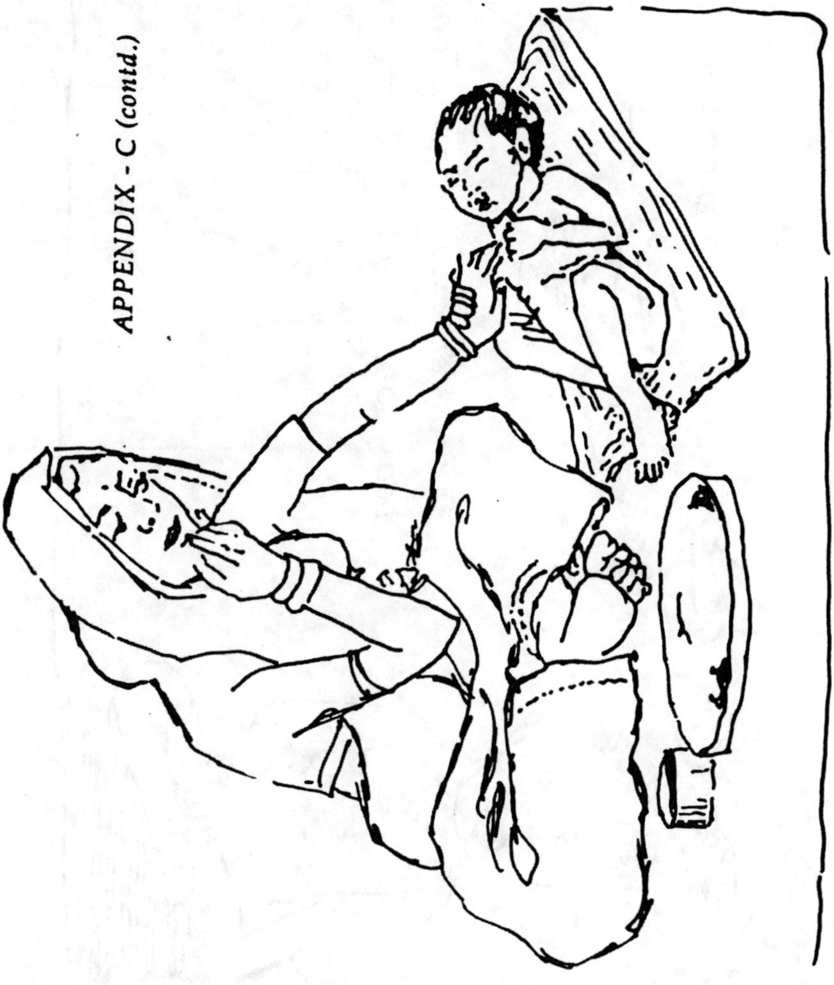

APPENDIX - C (contd.)

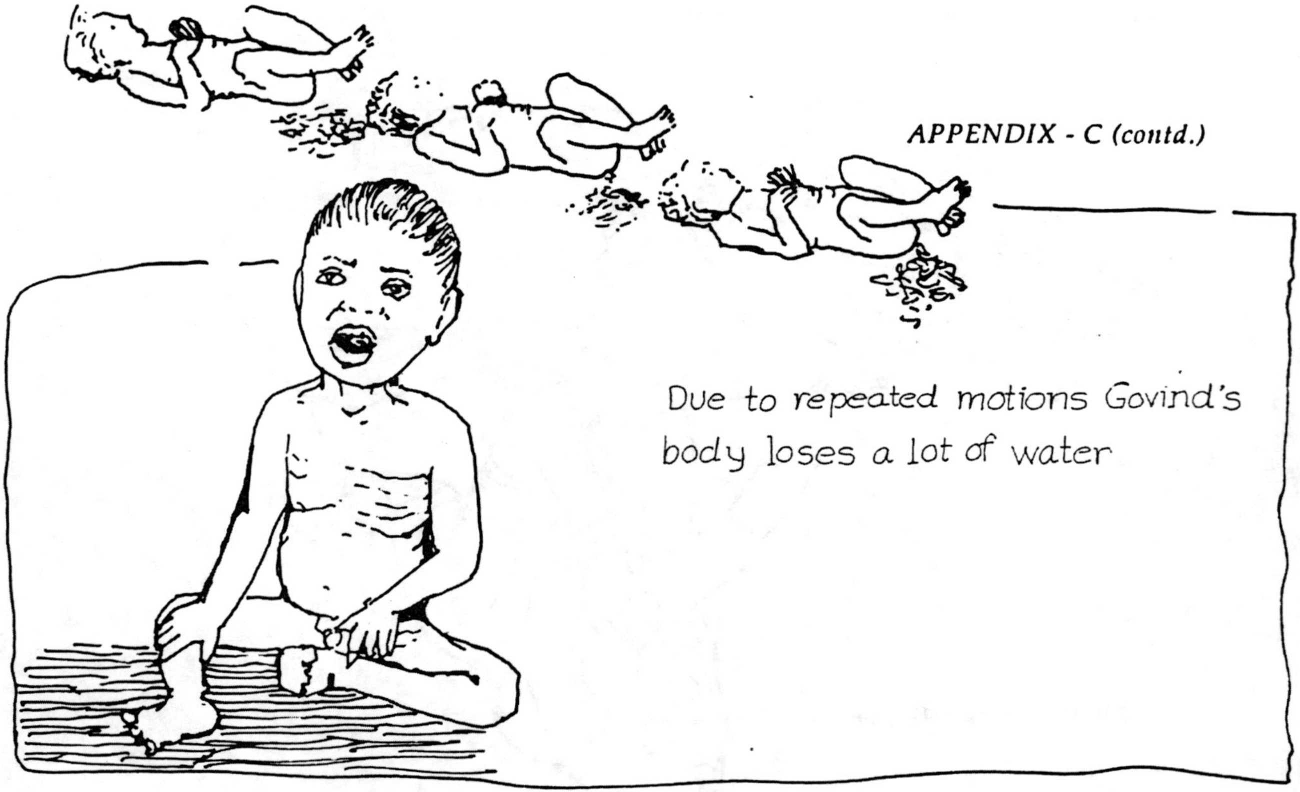

APPENDIX - C (contd.)

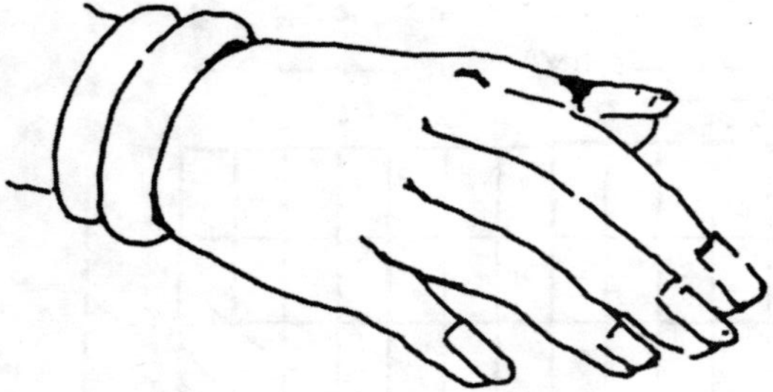

with these dirty hands Rama takes out a glass of water from the pot for Govind and also feeds him.

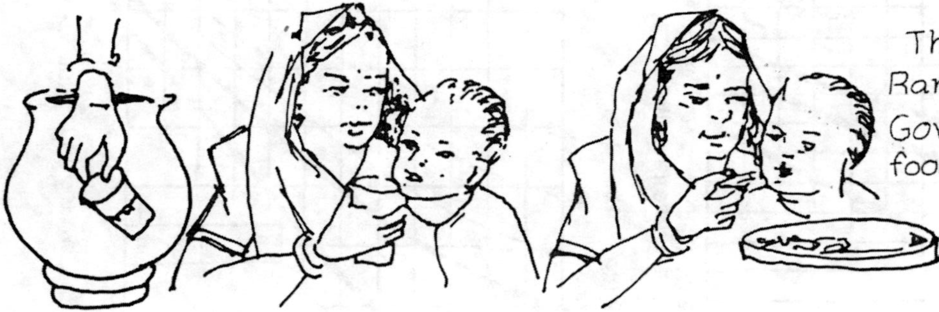

Thus the germs from Rama's finger nail reach Govind's stomach through food and water.

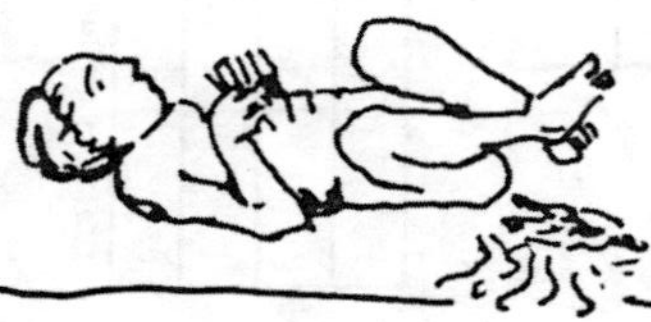

" GOVIND GETS DIARROHEA "

APPENDIX - D

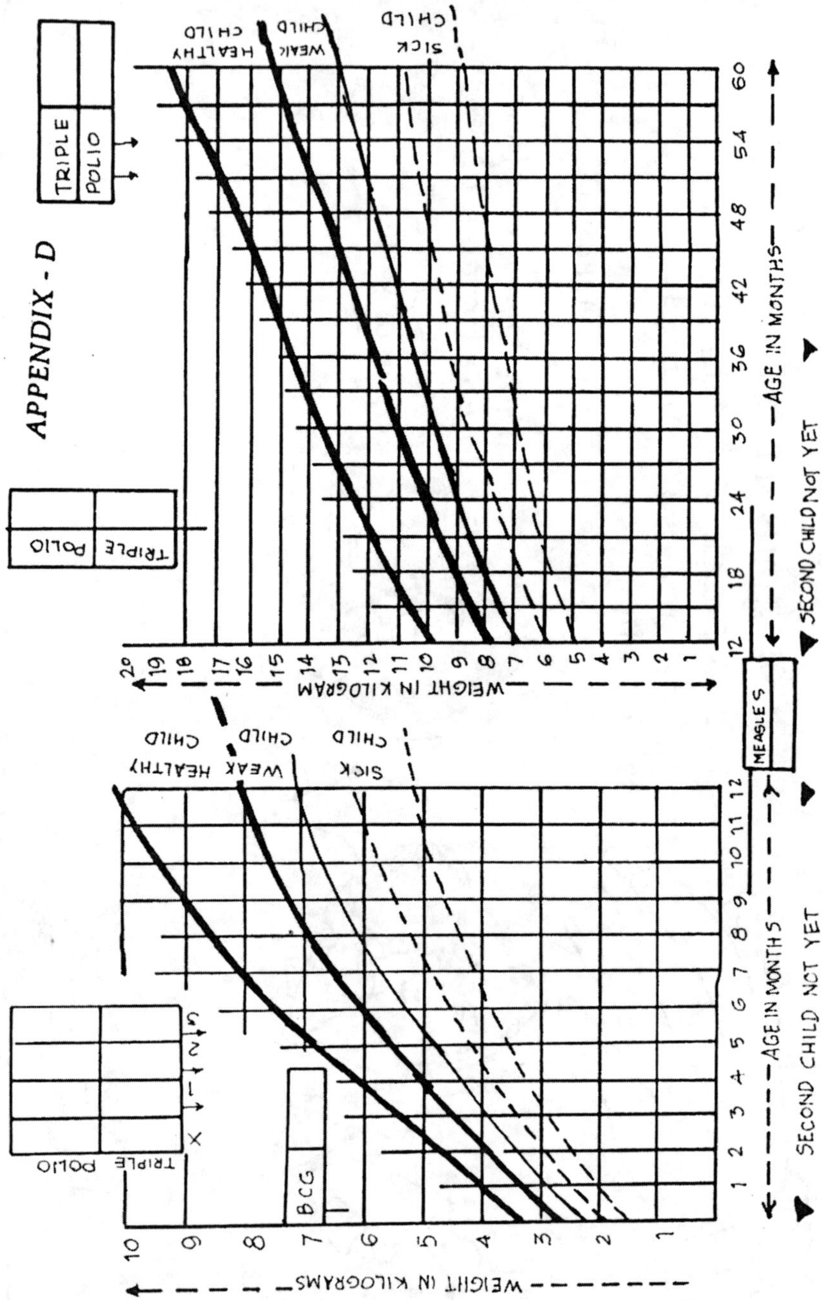
TRIPLE
POLIO
HEALTHY CHILD
WEAK CHILD
SICK CHILD
WEIGHT IN KILOGRAM
WEIGHT IN KILOGRAMS
AGE IN MONTHS
SECOND CHILD NOT YET
MEASLES
BCG

APPENDIX 'D' (Contd.)

IMMUNIZATION SCHEDULE

The following national schedule of immunization will be followed in ICDS project areas:

Age of Children		Vaccination
3-9 months	i)	Triple vaccine (DPT) against diphtheria, whooping cough and tetanus-3 doses at an interval of 1-2 months.
	ii)	Polio Vaccine-3 doses at an interval of 1-2 months.
	iii)	BCG vaccine (one dose only).
9-12 months		Measles vaccine—one dose (where available)
18-24 months	i)	Triple vaccine—(DPT)—Booster.
	ii)	Oral Polio—booster dose.
5-6 years	i)	Booster DT (Diphtheria & Tetanus Injection)
	ii)	First dose of typhoid monovalent or bivalent vaccine (Injection)
		After an interval of 1-2 months give second dose of typhoid vaccine (Injection)
Mothers		
Duration of pregnancy (1st)		
16-24 weeks		T.T. 1st dose
24-32 weeks		T.T. IInd dose

During subsequent pregnancy, this immunization is given only once if woman was immunized fully during Ist pregnancy if not then two doses are given as recommended.

Children

(a) The ages shown for the various immunizations are considered to be the most appropriate. However, it there is any delay in starting the first dose. The period may be adjusted accordingly. It should be the aim that the child before reaching one year of age should have received DPT, BCG and Polio vaccine and if available, measles vaccine. BCG, DPT and Polio can be given at the same time.

(b) When typhoid, DT or TT vaccine is being given for the first time two doses at an interval of 1-2 months, should be administered for desired effect.

APPENDIX 'E'

CODE BOOK/CARD DESIGN: 1 SUB: CHILD

Column	Information: Variable	Codes
1.	Group: V_1	Treatment-1 Control-2
2,3	Serial Number: V_2	Actual
4.	Card Number: V_3	1
5.	Age Group: V_4 (As in December 1986)	0-1 year-1 1+-3 year-2 3+-5 year-3
6-9	Height in cms. in Feb., '87: V_5 (One decimal point)	Actual
10-12	Weight in kg. in Feb., '87: V_6 (One decimal point)	Actual
13-16	Height in cms. in Apr. '87: V_7 (One decimal point)	Actual
17-19	Weight in kg. in Apr., '87: V_8 (One decimal point)	Actual
20-23	Height in cms. in Jun. '87: V_9 (One decial point)	Actual
24-26	Weight in kg. in Jun. '87: V_{10} (One decimal point)	Actual
27-30	Height in cms. in Aug. '87: V_{11} (One decimal point)	Actual
31-33	Weight in kg. in Aug. '87: V_{12} (One decimal point)	Actual
34-37	Weight/Height^2 x 100 as in Feb '87 (Three decimal places): V_{13}	Actual
38-41	Weight/Height^2 x 100 as in Apr '87 (Three decimal places): V_{14}	Actual
42-45	Weight/Height^2 x 100 as in Jun '87 (Three decimal places): V_{15}	Actual
46-49	Weight/Height^2 x 100 as in Aug '87 (Three decimal places): V_{16}	Actual
50-52	Haemoglobin as in Feb 87: V_{17} (One decimal point)	Actual

53-55	Haemoglobin as in Aug. '87: V_{18} (One decimal point)	Actual
56	Health/Nutritional Status in Feb. '87: V_{19}	Healthy-1 Weak-2 Sick-3 Dangerously sick-4
57	Health/Nutritional Status in Apr. '87: V_{20}	Healthy-1 Weak-2 Sick-3 Dangerously sick-4
58	Health/Nutritional Status in Jun. '87: V_{21}	Healthy-1 Weak-2 Sick-3 Dangerously sick-4
59	Health/Nutritional Status in Aug '87: V_{22}	Healthy-1 Weak-2 Sick-3 Dangerously sick-4
60	Religion: V_{23}	Hindu-1 Christian-2 Muslim-3 Any other-4
61	Caste: V_{24}	Non-caste-1 SC/ST Harijan-2 SC/ST other than Harijan-3 Upper Caste-4
62-63	Size of the Household: V_{25}	Actual
64-66	Food Consumption Units: V_{26} (One decimal points)	Actual
67	Type of Family: V_{27}	Nuclear-1 Joint-2
68	Mother's Educational Level: V_{28}	Illiterate-1 1 to 5 years-2 6 to 9 years-3 10 to 12 years-4
69	Father's Educational Level: V_{29}	Illiterate-1

		1 to 5 years-2
		6 to 9 years-3
		10 to 12 years-4
70	Occupation of Mother: V_{30}	House wife-1 Employed-2 earning Self employed earning-3
71	Occupation of Father: V_{31}	Hawker-1 Shop-keeper-2 Casual daily wage earner-3 Skilled Factory worker-4 Unskilled Factory worker-5 Contract Labourer-6 Badli Worker-7 Govt employee-8 Any other-Actual
72-74	Per-Capita Monthly Household Income: V_{32}	Actual
75-76	Mother's age: V_{33}	19-21 - 1 25-30 - 2 31-35 - 3

APPENDIX-F

CODE BOOK/CARD DESIGN: 2 SUB: MORBIDITY DATA

Column	Information: Variable	Codes	
1.	Group/V_1	Treatment-1	Control-2
2,3	Serial Number: V_2	Actual	
4	Card number/V_3	2	
5-10	Reported incidence of Diarrhoea in		
	Month	*Column No.*	
	March '87	(1) N.A.-0	
	April '87	(2) Once-1	
	May '87	(3) Twice-2	
	June '87	(4) Thrice-3	
	July '87	(5) Four Times-4	
	August '87	(6) Five Times-5	
		/V_4	
11-16	Reported incidence of Vomitting in		
	Month	*Column No.*	
	March '87	(7) N.A.-0	
	April '87	(8) Once-1	
	May '87	(9) Twice-2	
	June '87	(10) Thrice-3	
	July '87	(11) Four Times-4	
	August '87	(12) Five Times-5	
		/V_5	
17-22	Reported incidence of Low fever in		
	Month	*Column No.*	
	March '87	(13) N.A.-0	
	April '87	(14) Once-1	
	May '87	(15) Twice-2	
	June '87	(16) Thrice-3	
	July '87	(17) Four Times-4	
	August '87	(18) Five Times-5	
		/V_6	

23-28 Reported incidence of High fever in

Month	*Column No.*
March '87	(19) N.A.-0
April '87	(20) Once-1
May '87	(21) Twice-2
June '87	(22) Thrice-3
July '87	(23) Four Times-4
August '87	(24) Five Times-5

/V_7

29-34 Reported incidence of Skin diseases in

Month	*Column No.*
March '87	(25) N.A.-0
April '87	(26) Once-1
May '87	(27) Twice-2
June '87	(28) Thrice-3
July '87	(29) Four Times-4
August '87	(30) Five Times-5

/V_8

35-40 Reported incidence of Measles in

Month	*Column No.*
March '87	(31) N.A.-0
April '87	(32) Once-1
May '87	(33) Twice-2
June '87	(34) Thrice-3
July '87	(35) Four Times-4
August '87	(36) Five Times-5

/V_9

41-46 Reported incidence of Chicken Pox in

Month	*Column No.*
March '87	(37) N.A.-0
April '87	(38) Once-1
May '87	(39) Twice-2
June '87	(40) Thrice-3
July '87	(41) Four Times-4
August '87	(42) Five Times-5

/V_{10}

47-52 Reported incidence of Coughs and Colds in

Month	*Column No.*
March '87	(43) N.A.-0
April '87	(44) Once-1
May '87	(45) Twice-2

	Month	Column No.
	June '87	(46) Thrice-3
	July '87	(46) Four Times-4
	August '87	(47) Five Times-5
		/V_{11}

53-58 Reported incidence of any other disease in

Month	*Column No.*
March '87	(49) N.A.-0
April '87	(50) Once-1
May '87	(51) Twice-2
June '87	(52) Thrice-3
July '87	(53) Four Times-4
August '87	(54) Five Times-5
	/V_{12}

APPENDIX-G

CODE BOOK/CARD DESIGN: 3 SUB: MOTHER

Column	Information: Variable	Codes
1.	Group: V_1	Treatment-1 Control-2
2,3	Serial Number: V_2	Actual
4.	Card Number: V_3	3
5.	Age Group as in Dec. '86 V_4	19-24 - 1 25-30 - 2 31-35 - 3 Above 36 - 4
6.	Educational Status: V_5	Illiterate - 1 1 to 5 yrs - 2 6 to 9 yrs - 3 10 to 12 yrs - 4
7.	Occupational Status: V_6	House Wife - 1 Employed earning - 2 Self-employed earning-3
8.	Family Type: V_7	Nuclear - 1 Joint - 2
9-10	Household Size: V_8	Actual
11-13	Per-Capita Monthly Household Income: V_9	Actual
14	Total Score on Knowledge of Symptoms, care and management of sick child and prevention of Diarrhoea before H.E.P: V_{10}	Actual
15	Total Score on Knowledge of Symptoms, care and management of sick child and prevention of Diarrhoea after H.E.P: V_{11}	Actual
16	Total Score on Knowledge of Symptoms, care and management of	

	sick child and prevention of Measles before H.E.P.: V_{12}	Actual
17	Total Score on Knowledge of Symptoms, care and management of sick child; prevention of Measles after H.E.P.: V_{13}	Actual
18	Total Score on Knowledge of Symptoms, care and management of sick child; prevention of Chicken Pox before H.E.P.: V_{14}	Actual
19	Total Score on Knowledge of Symptoms, care and management of sick child; prevention of Chicken Pox after H.E.P.: V_{15}	Actual
20	Total Score on Knowledge of Symptoms, care and management of sick child; prevention of Anaemia before H.E.P.: V_{16}	Actual
21	Total Score on Knowledge of Symptoms, care and management of sick child; prevention of Anaemia after H.E.P: V_{17}	Actual
22	Total Score on Knowledge of Symptoms, care and management of sick child; prevention of Tetanus before H.E.P: V_{18}	Actual
23	Total Score on Knowledge of Symptoms, care and management of sick child; prevention of Tetanus after H.E.P.: V_{19}	Actual
24	Total Score on Knowledge of Symptoms, care and management of sick child; prevention of Scabies before H.E.P.: V_{20}	Actual
25	Total Score on Knowledge of Symptoms, care and management of sick child; prevention of Scabies after H.E.P.: V_{21}	Actual
26-27	Total Score on practice of care and management of sick child during childhood diseases Before H.E.P.: V_{22}	Actual

28-29	Total Score on practice of care and management of sick child during childhood diseases After H.E.P: V_{23}	Actual
30-31	Total Score on Knowledge of Advantages of Breast-feeding, weaning foods and weaning age Before H.E.P: V_{24}	Actual
32-33	Total Score on Knowledge of Advantages of Breast-feeding, weaning foods and weaning age After H.E.P.: V_{25}	Actual
33-35	Total Score on Attitude to Breast-feeding, weaning foods and weaning age Before H.E.P.: V_{26}	Actual
36-37	Total Score on Attitude to Breast-feeding, weaning foods and weaning age After H.E.P.: V_{27}	Actual
38-39	Total Score on Practice to Breast-feeding, weaning foods and weaning age Before H.E.P: V_{28}	Actual
40-41	Total Score on Practice to Breast-feeding, weaning foods and weaning age After H.E.P: V_{29}	Actual
42-43	Total Score Knowledge of Pre-Natal care Before H.E.P: V_{30}	Actual
44-45	Total Score Knowledge of Pre-Natal care After H.E.P.: V_{31}	Actual
46	Total Score Knowledge of Post-Natal care Before H.E.P: V_{32}	Actual
47	Total Score Knowledge of Post-Natal care After H.E.P.: V_{33}	Actual
48-49	Total Score Knowledge of advantages, methods and side-effects of Family Planning practices Before H.E.P.: V_{34}	Actual
50-51	Total Score Knowledge of advantages, methods and side-effects of Family Planning practices After H.E.P: V_{35}	Actual
52-53	Total Score on Attitudes towards Family Planning and contraception Before H.E.P.: V_{36}	Actual

54-55	Total Score on Attitudes towards Family Planning and contraception after H.E.P.: V_{37}	Actual
56	Blank	
57	Blank	
58-59	Total Score on Practice of personal hygiene (dental care, cleanliness of nails, hair, clothing) by mother before H.E.P.: V_{40}	Actual
60-61	Total Score on Practice of personal hygiene (dental care, cleanliness of nails, hair, clothing) by mother after H.E.P.: V_{41}	Actual
62	Total score on knowledge of balanced diet and nutrition for underfives before H.E.P.: V_{42}	Actual
63	Total score on knowledge of balanced diet and nutrition for underfives after H.E.P.: V_{43}	Actual
64	Total score on Attitudes towards women and female child before H.E.P.: V_{44}	Actual
65	Total score on Attitudes towards women and female child after H.E.P.: V_{45}	Actual
66	Total score on Attitudes to Health professionals and Services before H.E.P.: V_{46}	Actual
67	Total score on Attitudes to Health professionals and Services After H.E.P.: V_{47}	Actual
68	Total score on Knowledge of Health services in neighbourhood and city before H.E.P.: V_{48}	Actual
69	Total score on Knowledge of Health services in neighbourhood and city after H.E.P.: V_{49}	Actual
70	Total score on Knowledge of Immunization schedule and advantages before H.E.P.: V_{50}	Actual
71-72	Total score on Knowledge of Immunization schedule and advantages After H.E.P.: V_{51}	Actual

APPENDIX-H

CARD DESIGN: 4 SUB: RELIABILITY TESTING

Column/ Item No.	Information	Codes
1-2	Serial Number	Actual
3.	Age Group	19-24 - 1 25-30 - 2 31-35 - 3
4.	Occupational	House Wife - 1 Employed earning - 2 Self employed earning-3
5.	Family Type	Nuclear - 1 Joint - 2
6	Household Size	Actual
7-9	Per-Capita Monthly Income	Actual
10/1	Total Knowledge score: Diarrhoea	Actual
11/2	Total Knowledge score: Measles	Actual
12/3	Total Knowledge score: Chicken Pox	Actual
13/4	Total Knowledge score: Anaemia	Actual
14/5	Total Knowledge score: Tetanus	Actual
15/6	Total Knowledge score: Scabies	Actual
16-17/7	Total Practice score of Infant Feeding	Actual
20	Blank	
21-22/9	Total Attitude score of Infant Feeding	Actual
23-24/10	Total Practice score of Infant Feeding	Actual
25-26/11	Total Knowledge score of Pre-Natal Care	Actual
27/12	Total Knowledge score of Post-Natal Care	Actual

28-29/13	Total Knowledge score of Family Planning	Actual
30-31/14	Total Attitude score of Family Planning	Actual
32/15	Total Knowledge score of Nutritive diet	Actual
33-34/16	Total Practice score of Personal Hygiene	Actual
35/17	Total Attitude score on women and female child	Actual
36/18	Total Attitude score on Health Professional and Health Services	Actual
37/19	Total Knowledge score on Health Services available in neighbourhood and city	Actual
38-39/20	Total score on Knowledge of Immunization schedule and advantages	Actual
40	Time of test	Pre-1 Post-2

GLOSSARY

Advocate	:	It is an active, directive role in which a social information, for arguing the correctness of the client's (whether an individual or citizen's group) plea for help and for challenging the institution's indifference or negative response.
AIDS	:	Acquired Immuno Deficiency Syndrome.
Anganwadi	:	A neighbourhood centre for delivering Integrated Child Development Scheme services in a village/ urban slum.
Attitudes	:	Attitudes are evaluations of specific objects or conditions, *i.e.*, a judgement that an object or condition is "good or bad, desirable or undesirable, something to be approached or avoided....the object may be literally anything: a person, an event, an idea, a proposal for action, an action itself. People exhibit an attitude when they say that "government hospital services are bad".
BCG	:	Antituberculosis Vaccine.
Beliefs	:	Beliefs are judgements held with varying degrees of certainty that an object, process or action possesses a particular attribute. Like when the slum women say that "an infant should not be breastfed for three days immediately after birth".
Broker	:	In this role, a social worker links individuals and groups who need help but do not know where help is available to existing community services and resources.
DPT	:	Diptheria, Pertusis and Tetanus Vaccine.
Enabler	:	In this role a social worker helps individuals, groups or communities to articulate their needs, to

		clarify and identify their problems, to explore problem-solving strategies to select and apply a strategy and to develop their capacities to deal with their own problems more effectively.
Group	:	Group is a plurality of.individuals who are in contact with one another, who take one another into account, and who are aware of some significant commonality-an essential feature of a group is that its members have something in common and that they believe that what they have in common makes a difference.
Harijan	:	Literally, "Children of God", a term referring to 'jatis' formerly treated as low caste 'untouchables".
Infant Mortality Rate (IMR)	:	Annual number of deaths of infants under one year of age per 1000 live births. More specifically this is the probability of dying between birth and exactly one year of age.
Kaccha	:	A mud thatched, weak, not sturdy construction.
Khichadi	:	A soft gruel of rice and pulse.
Knowledge	:	Knowledge has been defined as the acquaintance with theoretical or practical understanding of some branch of science, art, learning or other area involving study, research, or practice and the acquisition of skills.
Low birth weight	:	Less than 2,500 grammes.
Maternal Mortality Rate (MMR)	:	Annual number of deaths of women from pregnancy related causes per 1000 live births.
NGO	:	Non-governmental Organization.
ORS	:	Oral Rehydration Salts.
ORT	:	Oral Rehydration Therapy.
ORT use	:	Percentage of all cases of diarrhoea in under five children treated with oral rehydration salts or an appropriate household solution.
PHC	:	Primary Health Centre.
Pucca	:	Of strong sturdy construction.
Ration Shop	:	A fair price shop under the public distribution system of the government where grains, kerosene, sugar and other consumer items are sold at subsidised

rates.

Self-determination: Implies that clients should be made aware that there are alternatives for resolving a personal or social problem they face. Further, it involves encouraging them to take decisions or choose the course of action(s) from available alternatives.

Skill : Is the ability to use knowledge effectively and readily in execution or performance.

TBA : Traditional Birth Attendant.

Under five Mortality Rate (U_5MR) : Annual number of deaths of children under five years of age per 1000 live births. More specifically this is the probability of dying between birth and exactly five years of age.

Values : Can be defined as generalized attitudes, beliefs, preferences that are adhered to rather consistently in judging particular objects which may be individuals, ideas, proposals for action or action itself. For instance, 'non-judgementality' on part of professional social workers, or the beliefs in people of 'serve thy neighbour'.

WHO : World Health Organization.

SELECTED BIBLIOGRAPHY

Unpublished Reports

Argade, S.C. (1987) "A study of the Urban Poor, M.S.W. Dissertation, Faculty of Social Work, M.S.U. of Baroda, Baroda".

Parikh, Y.O. (1982) "Income Consumption and Poverty Levels of Slum-dwellers in Baroda City, Ph.D. Thesis".

Tudu, S.J. (1982) "Social Intervention Role of Workers in Social Welfare Agency in Baroda, Ph.D. Thesis".

Published Reports

Anubhav, series (1988) "Experiences in Community Health Financing and the Health Needs of Poor Women and Children in India, The Ford Foundation, New Delhi".

Baroda Municipal Corporation (1976) "A report on the Slums of Baroda, Baroda".

Berman Peter (1990) "Ashish Gram Rachna Trust, Pachod, Maharashtra, Case Study No 4, Ford Foundation, New Delhi".

Berman Peter (1990) "SEWA—Rural, Jhagadia, Gujarat, Case Study No. 2, Ford Foundation, New Delhi".

Indian Council of Med. Research (1974) "Studies on Pre-school children, Technical Report No. 26, ICMR, India".

ICSSR and ICMR (1980) "Health for All: An Alternative Strategy, Indian Inst. of Edn, Pune".

Rajyaguru H.M. (1988) "Profile of Slums, Baroda Citizen's Council, Baroda".

World Health Organization (1976) "Protein Energy Malnutrition, Technical Report Series No. 584, WHO, Geneva".

World Health Organization (1976) "New Trends and Approaches in the Delivery of Maternal and Child Care Health Services Tech. Rep. Ser. No. 600, WHO Geneva.

World Health Organization (1983) "New Approaches to Health Education in Primary Health Care, Tech. Rep. Ser. No. 690, WHO, Geneva.

UNICEF (1984) "State of the World' Children Report, UNICEF Regional Office for South Central Asia, New Delhi, India".

UNICEF (1985) "Annual Report, UNICEF Regional Office for South Central Asia, New Delhi, India".

UNICEF (1987) "State of the World's Children Report, UNICEF Regional Office for South Central Asia, New Delhi, India".

UNICEF (1988) "Annual Report, UNICEF Regional Office for South Central Asia, New Delhi, India".

UNICEF (1989) "Annual report, UNICEF Regional Office for South Central Asia, New Delhi, India".

UNICEF (1991) "Annual Report, UNICEF Regional Office for South Central Asia, New Delhi, India".

UNICEF (1991) "Child Survival and Population Growth, Oxford University Press, U.K., U.S.A. "India".

UNICEF (1992) "State of the World's Children Report, UNICEF Regional Office for South Central Asia, New Delhi, India".

Miscellaneous

Balgopal R. *et al.* (1970) "Morbidity and Mortality in Pre-school Children" in Report of the Seminar on the Pre-school Child, Indian Council of Social Welfare, Madras.

Bhan M.K. and Ghosh S. (1986) "Successful Growth Monitoring, Some Lessons from India, UNICEF Regional Office for South Central Asia, New Delhi, India".

Caldwell J.C. and Santow G. (1991) "Selected Readings in the Cultural, Social and Determinants of Health, Health Transition series No. 1, Health Transition Centre, Australia.

Dept. of Child Development, Faculty of Home Science, M.S.U. of Baroda (1982) "Guidelines for Tribal Functionaries for Conducting Health, Nutrition and Family Planning Programme Ch.2.

Dept. of Human Development and Family Studies M.S.U. of Baroda (1986) "Have Tool, Will Measure, Monograph Ed. by Saraswathi T.S. *et al.*"

Gopaldas T. (1986) "Nutritional Status of Some Selected Tribes of Western and Central India, A Paper presented at 19th Annual Meeting of Nut. Soc. of India, in Nov 86 at NIN, India."

Magrabi F.M. and Verma A. (1987) "House-hold Resources and their Changing Relationships, Case Studies in Gujarati, India, International Agricultural Publications No. 3, Univ. of Illinois, Urbana-

Champaign."

The Economic Times Oct. 17 (1981) by Chandrashekkar M.R."

Times of India (1983) "Status of the Urban Poor Children in a Daily Newspaper published from New Delhi, India."

Trainers' Workshop on Qualitative Research Methods in Health Research (1991) "Background material compiled by Dept. of Health Services Studies, TISS, Bombay, The Ford Foundation, New Delhi and Dept. of International Health—The John Hopkins University."

World Federation of Public Health Asso. (1985) "Information for Action: Issue Paper on Growth Monitoring, Prepared by UNICEF, U.S.A. p.8.

World Health Organization (1984) "Training Manual on Res. Methodology on Child Labour and Health, Prepared by Training Workshop on Methodology of Action Research on Child Labour Health, p.37."

Books and Journals

Algyris C. (1979) *Intervention Theory and Method—A Behavioural Science View,* Addison-Wesley Publishing Co. Inc.

Alleyne G.A.O. *et al.* (1976) *The Assessment of Nutritional Status, Protein Energy Malnutrition,* Edward Arnold Publishers Ltd. London, Ch. 8,9.

Attkisson C.C and Broskowski A (1978) *Evaluation and the Emerging Human Need Concept* in Evaluation of Human Service Programs, Academic Press, New York p. 24.

Babbie Earl (1979) *The Practice of Social Research,* Belmont, Calif: Wadsworth.

Baer B.L. and Federico R. (1978) *Educating the Baccalaureate Social Worker,* Cambridge M.A.: Ballinger p. 92.

Bartlet H.M. (1970) "Analysing Social Work Practice by Fields, National Asso. of Social Workers New York."

Beedlove J.L. (1972) "Theory Development as a Task for the Evaluator" in *Evaluation of Social Intervention,* Ed. by Mullen E.J. *et al.*, Jossey-Base Inc. p. 55-70.

Berman Peter (1991) "Health Economics, Health Financing and the Health Needs of Poor Women and Children in India", The Ford Foundation, New Delhi."

Bhat C.M. and Dahia S. (1985) "Nutrition Status of Pre-school Children in Gangwa village of Hissar Dist. *Ind.J. Nutr. Diet et. 22.*

Blalock M.H. (1960) *Social Statistics,* McGraw Hill Book Co. Inc. N.Y. · Toronto, London.

Busi B.R. *et al.* (1987) "Food, Dietary Intake and Feeding Practices in Urban Slums of Visakhapatnam" *Ind.J.Nutr. Diet et.* Vol. 24 No. 6.

Butt H.W. (1980) "Indo-Dutch Project for Child Welfare" in *Profile of the Child in India* Ed. by Barnbas A.P. *et al.*, Ministry of Social Welfare, Govt of India.

C. Gopalan *et al.* (1982) *Nutrition Value of Indian Foods,* NIN and ICMR Hyderabad, India.

Carter G.W. (1960) "Measurement of Need" in Social Work Research, The University of Chicago, Chicago.

Central Committee on Health and Nutrition (1982) "Integrated Child Development Scheme: Information Document", AIMS New Delhi.

Central Institute of Res. and Trg. in Public Co-operation (1975) "Child Nutrition in Perspectives on the Child in India p.43-56.

Central Tech. Committee on Health and Nutrition (1986) "Integrated Child Development Scheme: Monitoring and continuing Education System", AIIMS, New Delhi.

Chakravarty A. (1958) "Morbidity in Children" in *Ind.J. and Child Health* Vol. 6 No. 2.

Champion D.J. (1981) *Basic Statistics for Social Research,* Macmillan Publishing Co. Inc. N.Y."

Choudhary S.N. (1980) "Child In Need Institute" in *Profile of the Child in India,* Ed. by Barnbas A.P. *et al.*, Ministry of Social Welfare, Govt. of India.

Chow N.W. (1984) "Poverty in an affluent City" in Report of 22nd International Congress, IASSW, Montreal, Canada.

Chowdhury M. and Rao K. (1983) "Nutritional Status of Pre-School Children and the Associated Factors, *Ind.J.Nutr. Dieter.* 20 (1).

Compton B. and Galaway B. (1984) "Social Work Processes, Dorsey" Press, Illinois, p.11.

Crew F.A.E. "Health, its Nature and Conservation", Pergamon Press, London.

Currimbhoy Z. and Phadake P. (1983) "Survey of Anaemia in Children in Bombay, Ind.J. of Child Health, Vol. 12, No. 8."

Dean J.G. *et al.* (1978) "Health Visitor's Role in Prediction of Early Childhood Injuries and Failure to Thrive" in *Child Abuse and Neglect* Vol. 2p. 8.

Djurfeldt and Lindberg (1975) *Pills Against Poverty: A Study of The Introduction of Western Medicine in a Tamil Village,* Curzon Press, India.

Dugdale A.E. (1971) "American J. of Clin. Nutri 24, 174."

Elmendorf L and Isley R.B. (1982) "Role of Women in Water Supply and

Sanitation", *World Health Forum,* Vol. 3, No. 2, WHO Geneva.

Fineman S. (1985) "Intervention Research and Stress Theory in Social Work Stress and Intervention", Gower Publications U.K. p.14-7."

Friedlander W.A. *Introduction to Social Welfare,* Prentice Hall of India Pvt. Ltd. New Delhi."

Gandhi V.K. (1963) "Morbidity and Mortality in Children" *Ind.J. of Child Health,* Vol. 12. No. 12."

Gist N.P. (1957) "Ecology of Bangalore, India; An East-West Comparison" in *Social Forces,* 35: 355-65."

Gopal A.K. (1980) "Comprehensive Rural Health Project, Jamkhed" in *Profile of the Child in India,* Ed. by Barubas A.P. *et al.*, Ministry of Social Welfare, Govt. of India.

Gray J. *et al.* (1976) "Perinatal Assessment of Mother-Baby Interaction" Child Abuse and Neglect: The Family and the Community, Cambridge, Mess Ballinger.

Joshi S. (1986) "Multi-disciplinary Approach to Community Problems" in Social Work, M.S. University of Baroda, Vadodara, India: p.45.

Kahn A.J. (1954) "The Nature of Social Work Knowledge" in *New Directions in Social Work* ed. Cora Kasius, Harper and Row, New York p. 6.

Kakkar D.N. (1987) *The Concept of Nutrition Field Monitoring An Assessment* Ed. by Gopaldas T. and Seshadri S., Oxford Univ. Press, New Delhi.

Kakkar S. (1987) "Nutritional Status of Pre-school Children in rural Hisar" *Ind. J. of Nutri Dietet* Vol. 24 No. 7 204-208.

Karkal M. (1991) "Health and Health Services in India" in *Primary Health Care* ed. by Yesudian C.A.K. TISS, Bombay 1: 12-31.

Khan A.J. (1960) "The Design of Research" in *Social Work Research,* The Univ. of Chicago, Chicago.

Kochar V. (1991) "Social Techniques for Primary Health Care" in *Primary Health Care* ed. by Yesudian C.A.K. TISS, Bombay 6: 90-101.

Krishnamurthy K.G. (1986) "Theoretical Considerations for Developing Indicators for the Measurement of Child Survival and Development" in *Monitoring Survival and Development of the Young Child* ed. by Bose A.B., NIPCCD, New Delhi, 1:3-12.

Lobo M. "Working with the Parents and the Community for the under-priviledged Pre-school Child" *in the Child and The community Ind. Asso. Pre-School Education,* Delhi, India.

Madan T.N. (1987) "Community Involvement in Health Policy: Socio-Cultural and Dynamic aspects of Health Beliefs" *Social Science and*

Medicine 25, 6: 615-620.

Millikan M.F. (1959) "Inqniry and Policy: The Relation of Knowledge to Action" in *The Human Meaning of Social Sciences* Ed. by Lerner D. Meridian Books New York.

Mullen E. and Dumpson J. (1972) *Evaluation of Social Intervention*, Jossey Bass Inc. Publishers.

Murthy N. (1986) "Development of a Multi-Level Child Monitoring System" in, *Monitoring Survival and Development of the Young Child* Ed. by Bose A.B:., NIPCCD, New Delhi, India.

Olmstead M.S. (1956) *The Small Group*, Random House, New York p.21-2.

Park J.E. and Park K. (1985) *Textbook of Preventive and Social Medicine*, Published by M/S. Banarsidas Bhanot, Jabalpur, India Ch. 2, 5, 11."

Pathak M. *et al.* (1985) "Perceived Morbidity, Medically Defined Morbidity Population Typology and Its Relevance in Planning for Health Services", Health and Population, *Journal of NIHFW*, New Delhi Vol. 8, No. 1, 12-18.

Patel A.S. and Lulla B.P. (1968) *Preparing a Thesis Proposal: A Handbook of Thesis Writing*, Acharya Book Depot, Baroda, India.

Pebley A.R. (1984) "Intervention Projects and the Study of Socio-economic Determinants of Mortality" *Population and Develop. Review, Suppl.*, to Vol. 10, The Population Council, N. York.

Pincus A. and Minahan A. (1973) "The Nature of Social Work Practice" in *Social Work Practice: Model and Method*, F.E. Peacock Publishers Inc. Illinois, U.S.A.

Polansky N.A. (1960) *Social Work Research*, University of Chicago, Chicago.

Powers G.T. *et al.* *"Practice Focused Research, Integrating Human Service Practice and Research*, Prentice Hall Inc, New Jersey."

Ramaiya K. and Kumar R. (1977) "Abstracts of Selected Research Studies in Child Health and Nutrition" Part I and II, Unit Tata Inst. of Soc. Sciences, Bombay.

Ramachandran P. (1970) "The Slums: A Note on Fact and solution with Special Reference to Bombay" in *Slums and Urbanisation* Ed. by Desai A.R. and Pillai D.S., Popular Prakashan, Bombay.

Rao K.V. and Singh D. (1970) *American J of Clin. Nutri.*, 23, 83.

Reid W.J. and Shyne A.W. (1969) *Brief and Extended Case Work*, Columbia Univ. Press, N. York.

Ripple Lilian (1960) "Problem Identification and Formulation" in *Social Work Research*, University of Chicago Press, Chicago.

Rossi P.H. and Freeman H.E. (1982) *Evaluation: A Systematic Approach*,

II edition, Sage Publications, Beverley Hills p.33.

Sathyamala C. *et al.* (1986) *Taking Sides: The Choices Before the Health Worker,* ANITRA (Asian Network for Innovative Training Trust) Publication, Madras, India.

Schneider C. *et al.* (1976) "A Predictive Screening Questionnaire for Potential Problems in Mother Child Interaction" *Child Abuse and Neglect: The Family and the Community,* Cambridge, Mass Ballinger Ch. 20.

Scrivens E. *et al.* (1985) "Measuring the Impact of Health Interventions: A Review of Available Instruments" *Effective Health Care,* Vol. 2, No. 6. 147-258.

Seal K.C. (1986) *Core Indicators for Monitoring Child Survival and Development of the Young Child* ed. by Bose A.B., NIPCCD, New Delhi 2: 15-34.

Seshadri S. and Saiyed F. (1987) "Nutrition and Health Edu. in the ICDS for Tribal Urban Households", *Household Resources: Case Studies in Gujarat, India* Ed. by Magrabi F.M. and Varma A. Univ. of Illinois Urban Champaign.

Shah. P.M. and Shah K.P. (1980) "Integrated Mother Child Health-Nutrition, Project, PHC, KASA" *Profile of the Child in India,* Ed. by Barnbas A.P. *et al.*, Ministry of Social Welfare Govt. of India.

Simons H. (1986) *Persuasion: Understanding, Practice and Analysis",* 2nd ed. Random House, New York p. 22-3.

Sohoni N.K. (1988) "Monitoring As a Means Towards Child Growth *Future* 24-25, UNICEF in Asia, N. Delhi.

Standard K. and Kaplun A. (1983) "Health Education: New Task; New Approaches, WHO Chronicle 37 (2)."

Stanfield J.P. (1976) "Principle of Nutrition Education *Proc. Nutri. Soc.* 35, 131.

Sukhatme P.V. (1978) "Assessment of Adequacy of Diets at Different Income Levels, Economic and Political Weekly, Vol. 13, Nos. 31, 32, 33."

Susskind E. and Klein D. (1985) "Multi-Paradigmatic Approach in Community Research, Methods, Paradigms and Applications", Preager Special Studies p.10.

The Open University (1980) "Intervention Block 4 units 9, 10, 11, 12", Open Univ. Press Milton Keynes p. 20-38.

Thomas E.J. (1984) *Designing Interventions for the Helping Professions,* Sage Publications, Beverley, Beverley Hills."

Tripody T. *Evaluative Research for Social Workers,* Englewood Cliffs,

Prentice Hall, N. Jersey.

Twaddle A.C. and Hessler R.M. (1977) *A Sociology of Health,* St. Lois, Mosby."

Vasantha K.N. (1980) "Tamilnadu Pre-school Project", *Profile of the Child in India,* Ed. by Barnbas A.P. *et al.*, Ministry of Social Welfare Govt. of India.

Vir S. (1987): "School Children and Community Health", *Future* 22-23 UNICEF in Asia, N. Delhi.

William L. Hays (1963) *Hypothesis Testing and Interval Estimation* in Statistics, Holt, Rinehart, Winston Publication.

Yesudian C.A.K. (1991) "Primary Health Care", Tata Inst. of Soc. Sciences, Bombay.

Zastrow C. (1990) "Introduction to Social Welfare—Fourth" ed., Wadworth Publishing Co., California, U.S.A.

INDEX